My Promise

My Promise

One Woman's Journey of Healing from Breast Cancer

Corinna Alandt

This book is dedicated to women who are confronting a diagnosis of breast cancer. May this book help you on your journey to devine health.

Contents

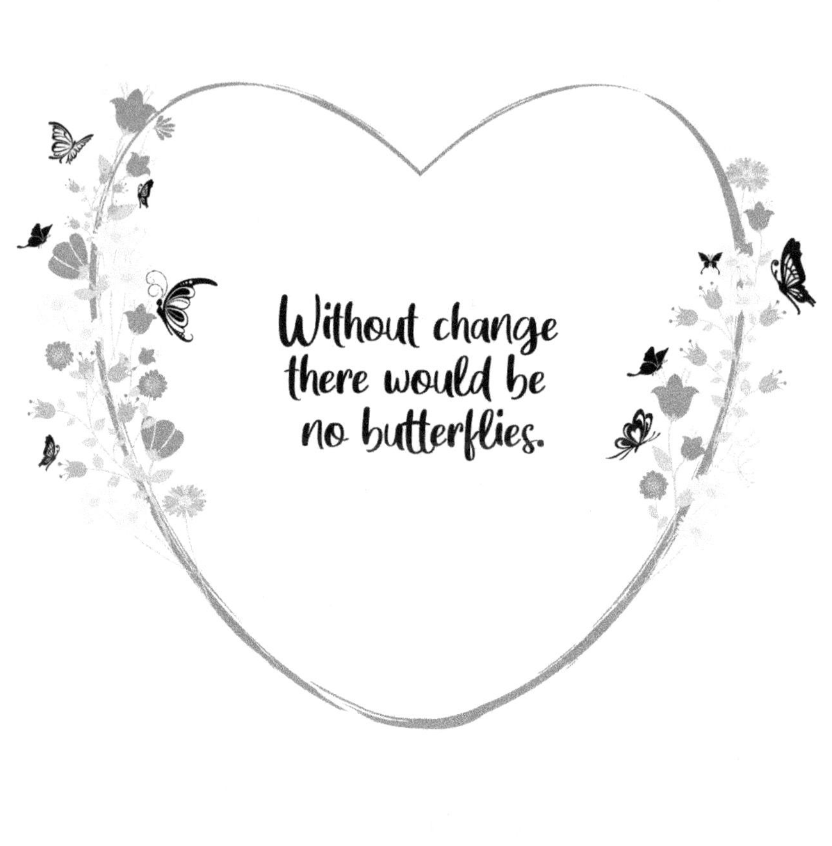
Without change
there would be
no butterflies.

Acknowledgements

Words will never be enough to thank my tribe of family, friends, surgeons and healers. I will treasure every note, call, text and home visit, but most importantly your prayers, which worked, and for that I am forever grateful.

A special acknowledgement to my husband, Robert—the year of cancer healing put our marriage vows of "in sickness and health" and "for better or worse" to the test. You are my rock, my confidant, my everything. I simply could not have asked for a better soul mate and partner during my healing journey. You are my light—one of the things that stuck with me and always will were your words when I looked back on 2019. I said 2019 was when I had cancer and you immediately said, "No, this is when you healed from cancer and changed your life so we can have another 40 plus years together." The depth of my love for you grew stronger this year than I thought was ever possible. April 2019 was our 20th wedding anniversary year, which we postponed celebrating. I am so looking forward to our new beginning and celebrating us in 2020! One quote you always said to me on a daily basis that kept me strong was "Tough times don't last—tough people do!"

To my children, Amanda and Mitchell—you are the reason I breathe. I will love you until the ends of the earth. You are my heart and soul. I am so proud to be your mother. Thank you for believing in me. You both were a light at the end of this journey. Our summer 2019 memories will be my favorite of all time. When I was healing, my days were spent thinking of this amazing family trip. *No one else will ever know the strength of my love for you, you are the only ones who know what my heart sounds like from the inside.*

To my rescue pooch Teddy Bear—You were always by my side, letting me spoon you, comforting me, licking my tears during my healing journey. Who recused whom nine years ago? I am the lucky one! *In a perfect world every home would have a dog, and every dog would have a home.*

To my best friend Claudia Narvaez—You are my soul sister, the sister I never had, whom God brought to me over 30 years ago. Your prayers on your knees, answering late night calls, books, cards and unwavering love and faith are treasures to me. God knew I needed you and you showed up in every single way. *A good friend knows all of your stories; a best friend helped you write them!*

To Nancy Vandergriff, the lady who, at the young age of 18, became my mom—You are the most positive person I know. You never let your faith waiver and you called everyone in the state of Texas for their prayers. But the ones you and Bubba, my brother, sent me every day where the ones I relied on the most. God is within you both and I knew He would listen and deliver. I love you, Mom. How did God know that I needed you as my mom? *I love this quote—Strong as a Mother!*

Thank you to all my friends and family who sent me these uplifting quotes that I saved, knowing they would be a perfect addition to this story. Thank you to sweet Kelsey D for creating the beautiful artwork throughout the book. You are so talented!

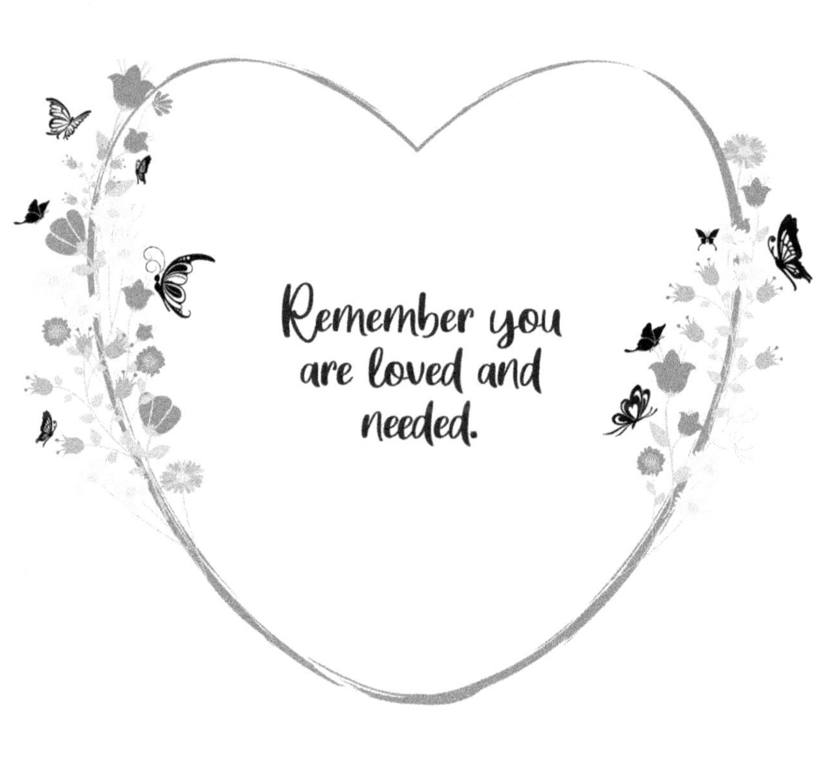

Remember you
are loved and
needed.

Foreword

We all face challenges in our lives. It's how we respond to these challenges that helps to define who we really are. Anyone who gets the opportunity to know Corinna Alandt comes away learning that among her many great qualities, she is a very compassionate, caring, loyal, intelligent, organized and determined individual. It is these qualities that she used to take on her challenge of breast cancer and I, as her husband, had a front row seat to watch them on full display each and every day. Never a person to take on the victim role, Corinna endeavored to read multiple books and writings on the subject as well as talking to a number of individuals to learn as much as she could about her disease to pursue the best treatments possible for her to not only overcome it, but to prevent it from ever recurring. In this book Corinna chronicles her journey for other women with a similar diagnosis to not only share her experiences with them, but to possibly help provide them some ideas to take control of their own treatment and to not blindly just accept what they might be told about their proposed treatment plan. I am very proud of Corinna for the way she took on this challenge and for documenting her journey so that other women confronted with the same challenge might benefit in some way from her experience by reading this book.

Robert Alandt

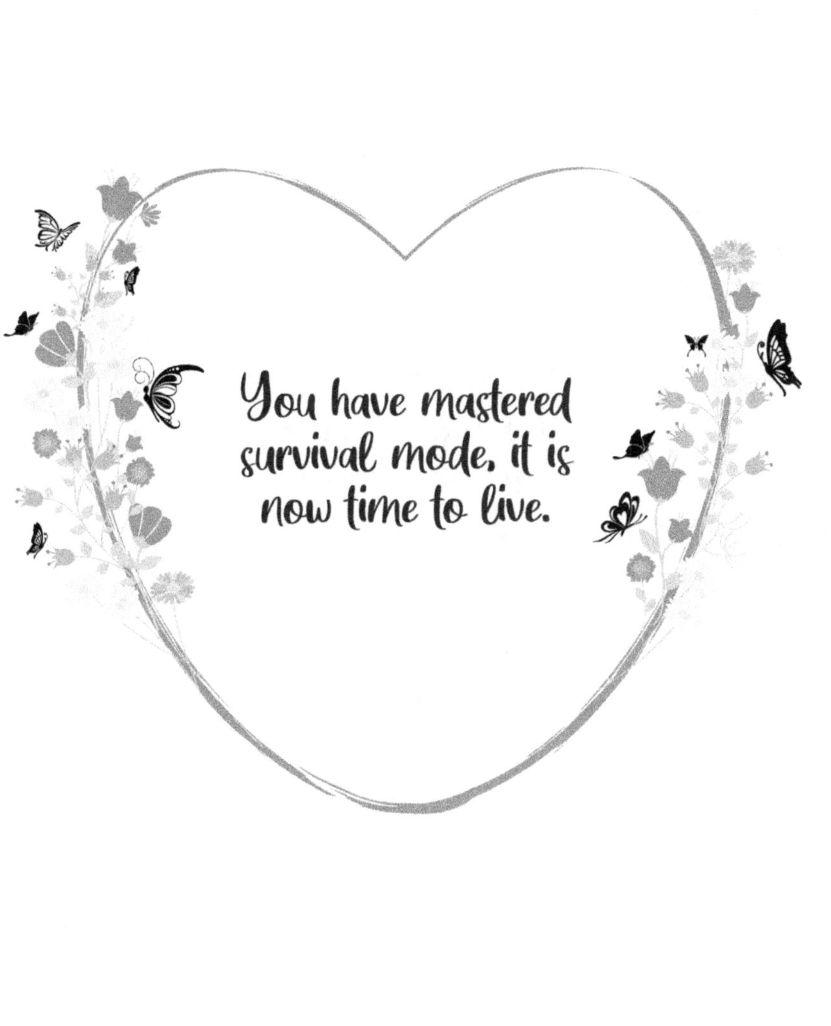
You have mastered
survival mode, it is
now time to live.

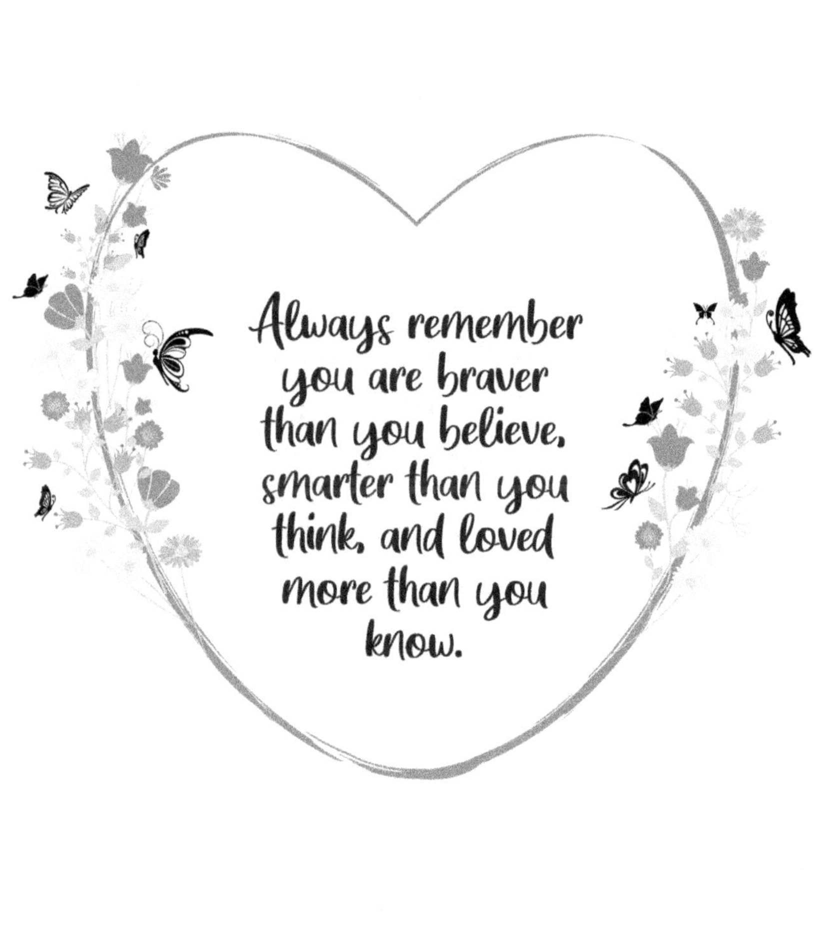
Always remember
you are braver
than you believe,
smarter than you
think, and loved
more than you
know.

This book is my promise to share my story of miracles and healing from breast cancer. If my story touches and helps ease the mind of one person, I have met "my promise."

My promise to God was that if he gave me a second chance at life and divine health, I would never take another day for granted and I would tell my story of miracles and healing to help spread the word that anything is possible when you have faith. I am blessed beyond measure for the health miracles I received, and I am confident that when you believe and put your trust in God miracles do happen! I am living proof.

I made many changes in my life after hearing the word *cancer*, which I will refer to often as the C word. I spent many countless days and hours reading and researching everything I needed to know about this disease. My story is about believing, having faith and sharing all that I've learned with someone who needs it as much as I did when I was first diagnosed. You are not alone as a breast cancer survivor. I am here to tell you that you are loved, there is hope and to always BELIEVE!

Let me begin by saying that I never thought "cancer" would be part of my vocabulary. What has been part of my vocabulary and my life are autoimmune disorders, depression and mental disorders—yep that's me, but cancer, absolutely not!

Prior to cancer I would have classified myself as a Type A+++ personality: striving for perfection in everything, sprinting to the finish line of every project or task and not taking any time to enjoy the journey along the way. Every work task, kid's party or social event I hosted was completed on time and in my eyes had to be "perfect." Not eating well, not sleeping enough, worrying like crazy, holding on to past hurt, simply not doing much of anything for self-care were the norm.

I thank God for my divine tap on the shoulder to slow down. I know in my heart that I would not have changed otherwise. Thank you, Lord, for this gift of life and gratefulness.

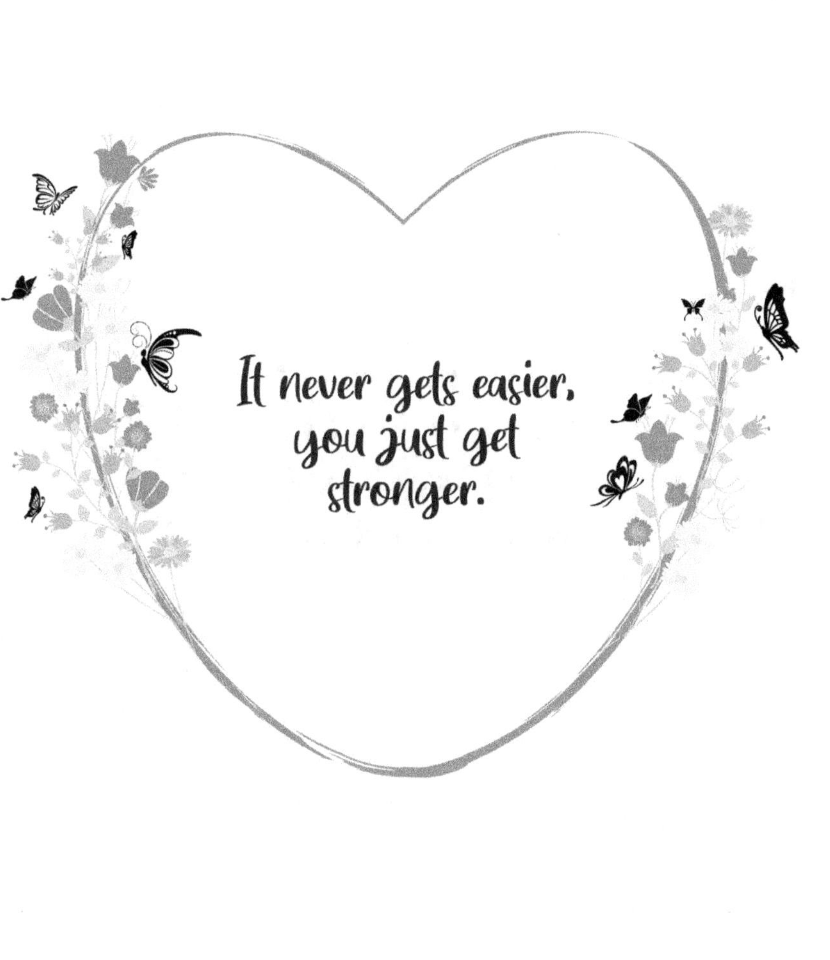
It never gets easier,
you just get
stronger.

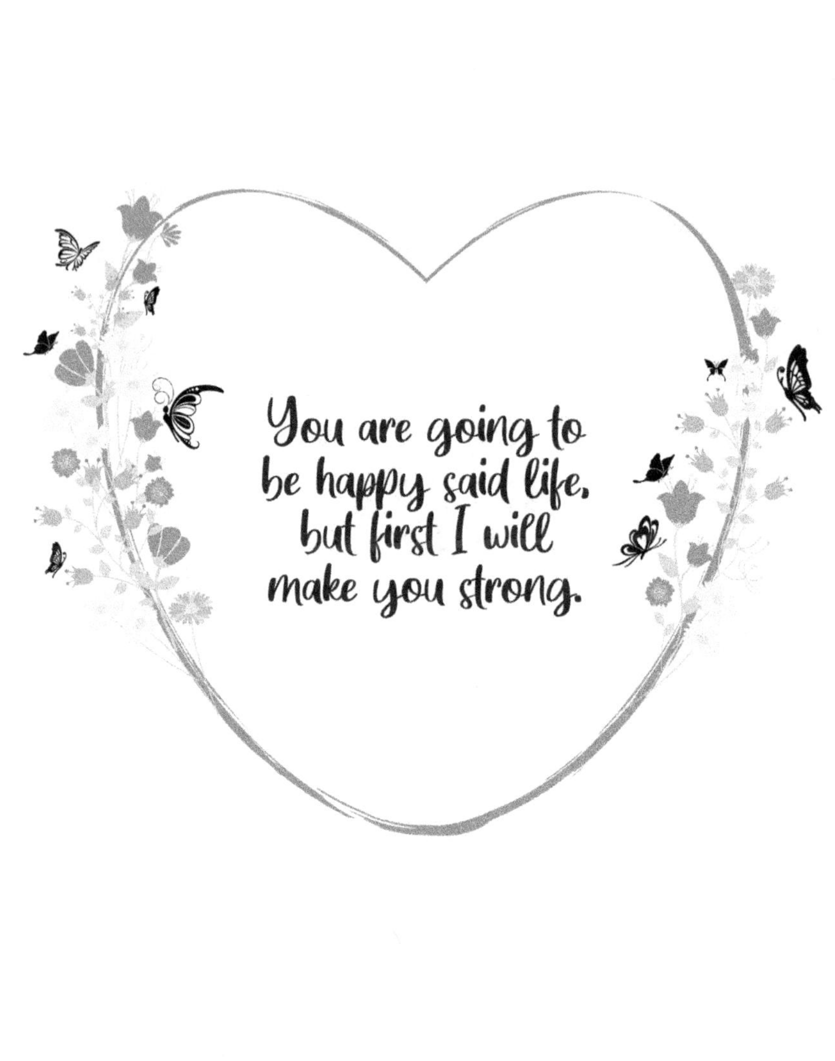
You are going to
be happy said life,
but first I will
make you strong.

Chapter 1: "I don't have time for this . . ."

Every January of every year for the past 14 years I have my yearly mammogram. January 2019 was no different. Everything was routine, quick and easy. I left the breast center clinic as usual, planning on a clear report to be sent in the mail and to schedule another appointment for the following year. A few days later I left for a business trip to Colorado. As with all business trips the days were packed with all-day meetings and evening work events. On the first day of the meetings, I noticed that I had three missed calls from the clinic that performed the mammogram. I had no time to call them back the first few days of the trip; however, after the sixth missed call I called them back by mid-week. The receptionist said the breast specialist would like to see me back for another test and asked when I could come in. This was the first time I was ever called back for a second test. My thoughts were, "I don't have time for this."

I flew home on a Thursday night, and on Friday at 9 am I had my follow-up appointment. This one was different. I was placed in an ultrasound room where a technician used an ultrasound machine on my left breast to continue to review the area that was "suspicious." My heart raced as they took what seemed like 50 images of a tiny area of my breast. The technician left the room and called in the doctor, who reviewed the images. The doctor informed me that she was recommending a biopsy of the area and I could come back the following Friday to perform the biopsy. I immediately told her I wasn't leaving the hospital until the biopsy was done that day. I told her I would have seven sleepless nights worrying about the images. She sent me home to grab my husband so he could drive me home after the procedure. When we returned, she called in another doctor to help with the biopsy. The biopsy technician numbed the area and said it wouldn't hurt. She was half right. It didn't hurt until after the numbing medication wore off and then the dull pain was a constant reminder that I must WAIT another three to four days to hear the results from the laboratory. The date that the test results were expected was the day I was meant to be celebrating my friend's 50th birthday. Again my thought was, "I don't have time for this!"

Those three days and nights of waiting were nerve wracking and I didn't sleep at all. Only my husband, my confidant, knew that the phone call was coming in. I am not sure he slept much either.

> *Key Message: Early detection is key. My lump was found on my annual mammogram.*

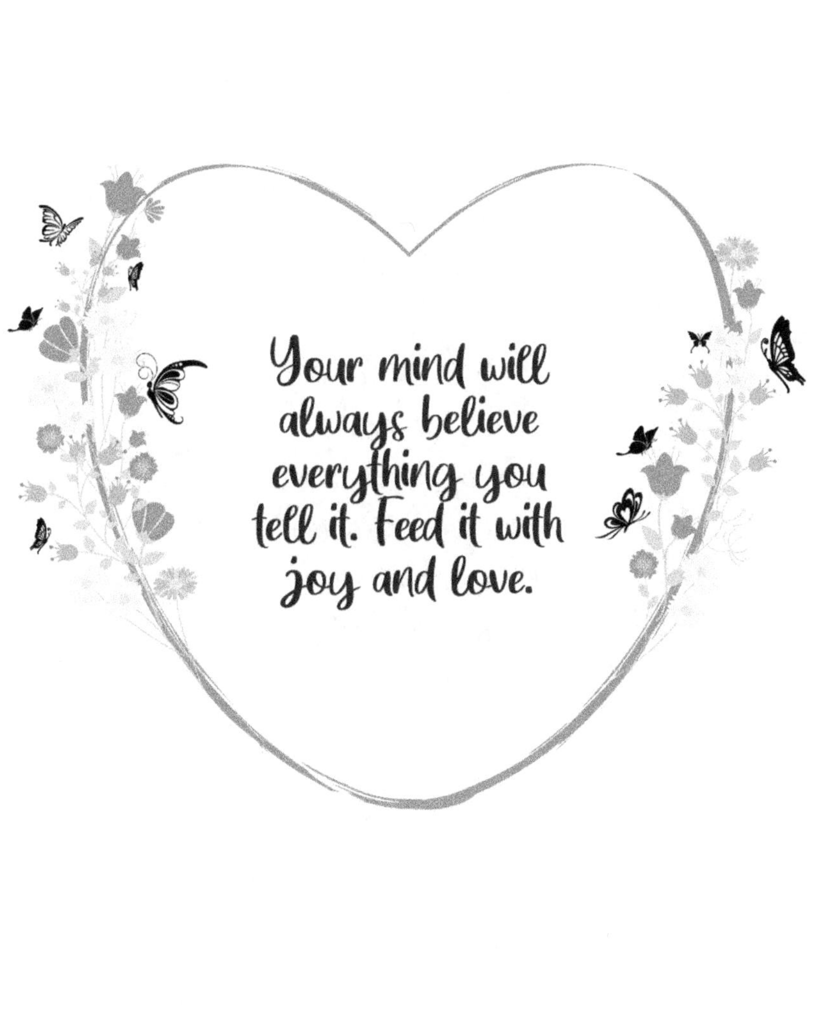

Your mind will
always believe
everything you
tell it. Feed it with
joy and love.

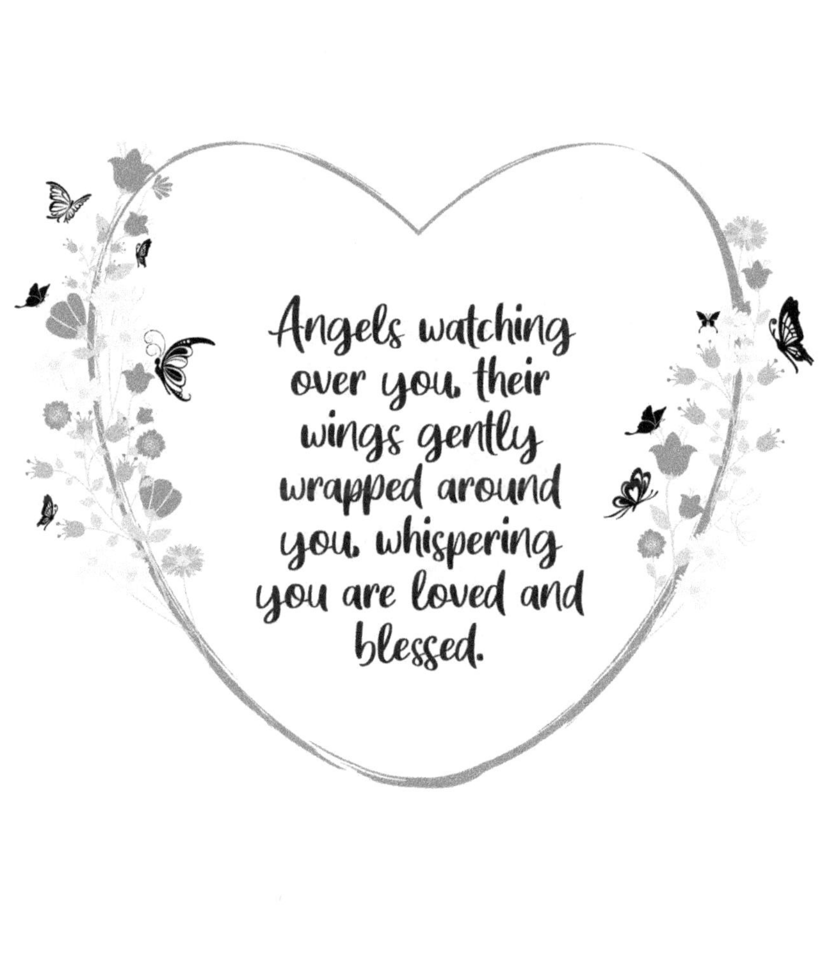
Angels watching
over you, their
wings gently
wrapped around
you, whispering
you are loved and
blessed.

Chapter 2: The call back and the C word

The day everything changed. I will never forget the day and time when the phone rang to share the results from the biopsy. I know where I was, what I was wearing, and yes, it was the same day as my friend's 50th birthday luncheon. I am grateful that the call came in after I was back at work. I saw the number on my phone and knew it was the breast center calling. I left my office and went into an empty office away from my work team so the conversation could not be overheard. I answered the phone and I heard the words I dreaded the most: "The results of your tests show you have breast cancer." The doctor proceeded to tell me that on Monday of the following week I would have a "team" of specialists who would meet with me and my husband to discuss the next steps. This hospital has a good reputation for treating breast cancer compassionately. I have dear friends who have been treated by them and have had great results.

I was in complete shock. I grabbed my things from my office, called my husband and asked that he come home. I had to tell my husband the news—not only will I never forget the call, I will never forget the look on my husband's face. This is the guy who has been my rock, my partner, my everything, and for the very first time in our marriage he looked scared. Neither of us cried, again both still in shock about what was to come next in this journey.

I can't remember if the second person I called was my mom or my best friend—it was a blur—but I needed them both desperately. I needed to cry, scream, swear (boy, did I swear) and ask for the kind of advice only a mom and a BFF can give. I also needed advice on when to tell my two children, aged 24 and 18. Both have busy lives and they didn't need my drama to deal with as well. Both kids were out of the house so I had time to think of the message I would share with them. The love and support from my mom and my best friend were overwhelming. I cry now thinking about those late-night calls. All three of us got on our knees and prayed—not a half-assed prayer but a gut wrenching, begging-for-a-miracle prayer. My mom is in Texas and my best friend is 30 miles from me, but I felt that they were in my bedroom with my pleading to our Lord. The next day my best friend delivered what she called a Dear Lord journal to me. She said she has one that she writes in every night: praying to the Lord, thanking the Lord and being grateful for his daily blessings. The first page of my new journal was her prayer to the Lord for me, the most touching message I have ever read. From the day she handed me my Dear Lord journal I have written in it every day, and when all the pages were filled I bought her a matching Dear Lord journal. I will continue to journal every single day. I didn't realize how much I missed journaling and how healing it is.

I had to trust God. I desperately felt I wanted to live. I had always been in control of my life, and now I had no control over my health or my future. I knew God was the only person who could provide me peace, comfort and help. I knew my faith, relationship and hourly conversations with God would be the most important part of my healing journey. I read so many Bible verses on healing—true miracles. I chose one verse that I repeated over and over hourly until I could calm my mind: "Through Jesus's stripes I am healed. Amen." I knew I had to make changes in my life, but deep down I knew God was the one who could save me. I'd had faith prior to the diagnosis, but this wake-up call brought me closer to Him than I have ever been.

What was next was trying to act normal at work and pretend that everything was fine when all I wanted to do was wake up from this nightmare. I started to read in the wee hours of the night. Let me tell you, Dr. Google is not your friend. I highly recommend not researching the topic of cancer on the internet. Many things are outdated and not accurate. My next move was to wait and meet with my medical experts on Monday.

> *Key message: A cancer diagnosis is terrifying. Find your small tribe on whom you can lean, cry to and share how darn scared you are until you know your next steps. First in your tribe should be God.*

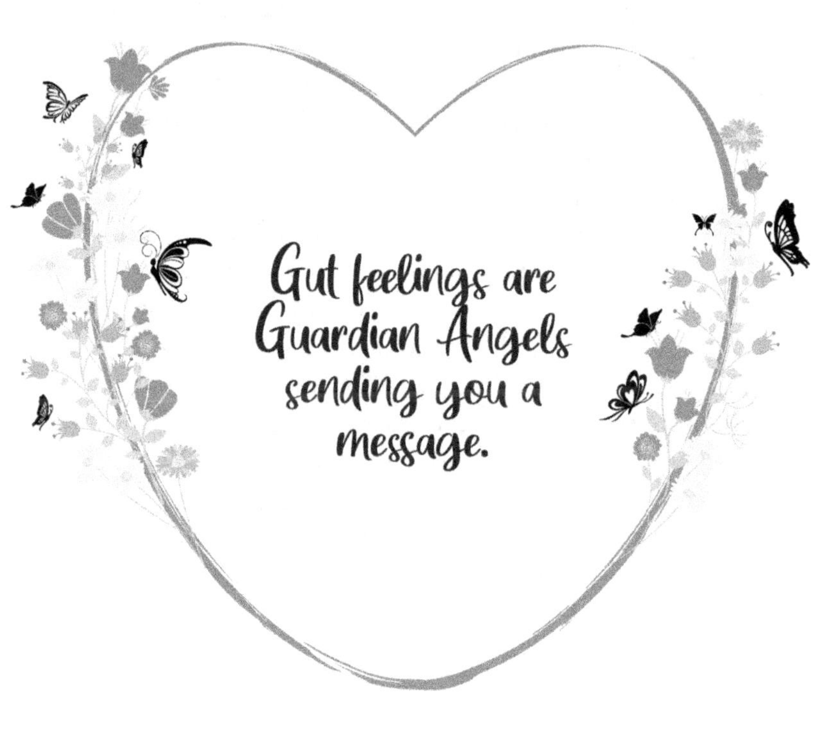
Gut feelings are
Guardian Angels
sending you a
message.

Chapter 3: You have choices—who knew!

The week after the call from the breast center was a blur. I didn't eat much because I thought everything that I put in my mouth would cause my cancer to grow. My mind raced, every moment thinking about how I would tell my kids, my family and my colleagues at work. I was nervous but also excited that I was about to meet the team that was being put together to discuss me, my breasts and the plan for my treatment. I had no idea what to expect but I was hopeful since so many before me had had a great experience with this local breast center.

My husband said he will never forget the looks of shock and bewilderment on the faces of other couples in the breast center waiting room. The doctors at the center kept reassuring me that they were there for me, however, I felt like I was a number, just another case they had seen thousands of times—rinse and repeat the standard treatment. I was introduced to "my team"—the surgeon, the radiologist and the medical oncologist—which I found out was the chemo doctor. I thought I was going to get physically sick listening to each of them speak about my next steps. Never once did they ask me what I thought. The surgery sounded horrific and I was given few options other than what I would consider a "butcher job." When my husband tried to ask questions he was brushed off. Each one of them felt the need to give my breast a physical exam—I'm not sure why; they had the results from the biopsy.

They proceeded to tell us that they classified my breast cancer as triple negative—one that could not be treated with an estrogen blocker medication, so radiation was a must and chemo should be strongly considered. They started quoting statistics on the survival rate of my type of cancer and had the balls to say to me, "At least your kids are older. You don't need to care for them anymore." EXCUSE ME?- I want grandkids to care for, and maybe great-grandkids. I was pissed off, nauseated and more nervous than ever after meeting "my team," who was to support me throughout this journey. Looking back and now having grace in my heart, I believe what they were trying to say was that my kids were out of the house and older so I could heal without worrying about them (this is my new view on people—thinking the best), but at that time I wanted to punch them all in the face. Guess what? I decided to FIRE "my team"— yes, my team of skilled doctors, highly regarded in my community. I still have PTSD from that team meeting but the decision to never return was the best decision I could have ever made. I prayed that night for answers on what I would do next.

The next day my wonderful and amazing OB/GYN called me out of the blue (I now consider it divine intervention) to say she'd seen the results of my biopsy and offered words of encouragement. It didn't dawn on me to reach out to her or that she would be copied on the biopsy results. What she offered me was priceless; she highly encouraged me to see a top surgeon who specialized in breast cancer at one the best teaching hospitals in northern California, which happened to be only a 20-minute drive from my home. She said that if she were in the same situation she would only trust this specific breast surgeon, who offered many options for treatments. From that moment on I knew that I had to form my own team of experts to help me through this journey. We are so programmed to believe that we should stay with our doctors and listen blindly to their advice. It was liberating to realize I had choices! I believe in my heart that God had used my OB/GYN to deliver the message he wanted me to hear, the first of many messages.

> *Key Message: Cancer does not grow overnight. You have time to research the best treatment options for you and to assemble the best team!*

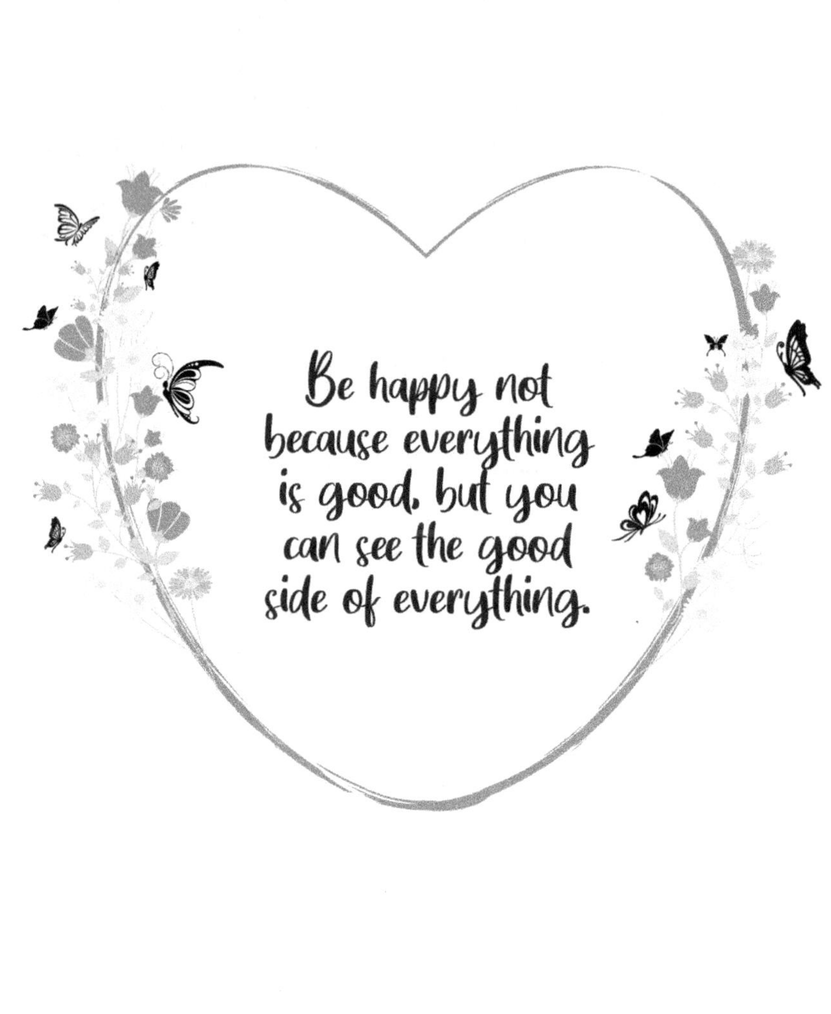

Be happy not
because everything
is good, but you
can see the good
side of everything.

Chapter 4: Making lemonade out of lemons

During this process I never once said, "Why me?" I knew why I had cancer. I was stressed out at my job working 16 hours a day, had an untreated autoimmune disorder, did not exercise and ate loads of sugar when I was stressed, not to mention holding on to past hurt and anger.

After speaking with my OB/GYN I was more energized than I had been since hearing of my diagnosis. I was able to book an appointment with my breast surgeon within days. My husband and I walked in expecting to be given a plan, "her plan," but instead she offered many options for my surgery. She was very self-assured—blunt but still compassionate. After my exam, she shared that since I was "very busty"—those were her words—I might benefit from a breast reduction. Not only could she remove the cancer from my left breast and take much more of the surrounding tissue, which would be beneficial, but she could bring in a plastic surgeon to provide a reduction on both breasts—"Unless," she said, "you like being a size E." I thought to myself, "Who the heck wants to be a size E? Maybe a porn star, but not me!" My husband and I both chuckled since we both knew that I had always wanted a breast reduction. I had been looking to get a reduction, but without the cancer diagnosis—God had different plans. I remember what my surgeon said: "You are making lemonade out of lemons!" From that moment on, I knew I was in amazing care and my next stop was to meet the plastic surgeon—a top one in the area—and coordinate the date for my surgery.

Two days later I met my plastic surgeon; what an amazing doctor he was, so kind and understanding. I had a feeling he had a special place in his heart for women who came to him while dealing with breast cancer rather than just getting larger and perkier breasts. He promised to take good care of me, and I knew he would. I told him that I was not planning on being in a "boob" contest, I just wanted him to do his best to have me wake up from the surgery. My doctor is such a perfectionist and reminded me that any woman who has surgery from him should be entering a boob contest.

The only downside with my new amazing surgeons was the wait. I had to wait almost 3.5 weeks to get on both their calendars for the surgery. At the time it felt like a lifetime; the cancer would grow and spread during those weeks of waiting. My surgeon assured me it doesn't happen that fast! My amazing, skilled doctors, to whom God had guided me, were worth the wait. Most people only have one surgeon for their breast surgery. I had two of the best in northern California working on me alongside each other. Following my meeting with the two surgeons, I was sent home to start on my mental healing journey and focus on self-care. I was not pressured to meet with a radiologist or a medical oncologist. What a difference from my first "team of experts." I did, however, have to undergo many tests to ensure that the cancer was only in my breast and had not spread, and to establish a baseline. Each test was terrifying. I was sent for a lung X-ray, bone scan, brain scan and liver scan. With each test I prayed they would be clear, and they were. After all the tests were completed it was time to share the news with the people who needed to know and who I needed to lean on. Leaning on others is not one of my strengths, a fault of mine I would need to change.

> *Key Message: Look for the good in your cancer message. I promise you will find it.*

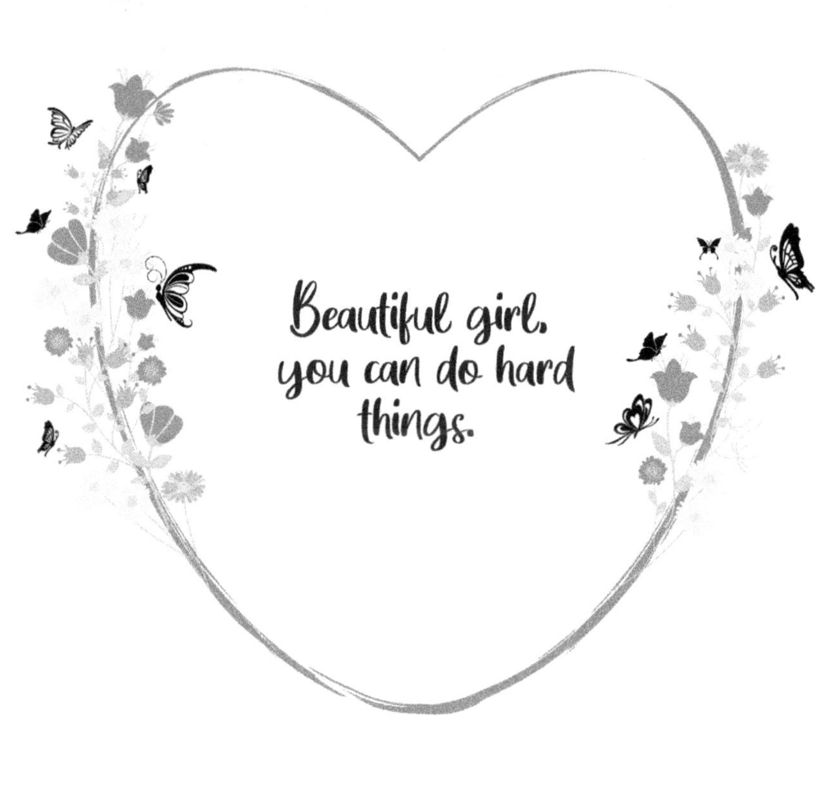
Beautiful girl,
you can do hard
things.

Chapter 5: Coming out

My surgery was coming up and I knew I had to tell more people other than my small circle of confidants. I needed prayers; I needed a miracle. After reading all of the information on triple negative breast cancer (TNBC) I was scared, my parents were scared, my brother was scared, my husband was scared, my best friend was scared. I searched to find any positive stories of long survival rates and there were few. I started reading uplifting stories of miracles, radical remission, self-cures for cancer through holistic care. Most importantly I read Bible verses of healing miracles. From the moment I left my surgeon's office I read everything I could, I prayed every moment I could and it was a lot. I prayed over my breast and begged God to not let this be TNBC. I prayed that my tumor would shrink away and when the surgeon went in they would find nothing (at this point a ridiculous thought, I know, but if you don't ask you may not receive).

I was pleading and that is when I made my promise to God; if he gave me a second chance at life and divine health, I would cherish every day and help others with my story. My parents live in Texas and I know my mother contacted everyone she knew and everyone at the local churches were praying for me. My best friend had her church praying for me. Whenever anyone asked what I needed I said prayers. I said, "Please don't say you will pray, *please pray hard for a miracle.*" Prayers are powerful and I knew very good people who served the Lord everyday had a good chance of him listening.

Although I'd told my daughter, who prayed for my healing, that I had cancer, she did not know that I may be dealing with TNBC. She was very scared. She stayed with me a few nights a week at my request; I needed her. I was scared that now she would have to put on her medical record that her mom had breast cancer. I now understand that less than 5% of breast cancer is hereditary. I know mine was not! I pray every day that this cancer stops with me and that no other women in my family or my friends have to hear those words.

My son at that time was in college and was not aware of my diagnosis. I could have used his prayers but it was more important to me that he focus on his first year of college. My goal was to tell him after the cancer was removed. That way I could say I *had* cancer and it had been removed. Boys cannot handle seeing their mother sick; at least that was my experience and rationale.

I had been with my company for 28 years, however, I'd only worked for my new boss for less than four months. Imagine telling your male boss, whom you are trying to impress in the first months of working together, that you have breast cancer and need to take a medical leave of absence. I was worried, but I couldn't have asked for a more understanding person. One of the things he said that made all the difference in the world was, "You have been here for twenty-eight years. You have earned the right to go and take care of yourself without worrying.

You have built a great team. Let them take over. They will want nothing more and this will be their gift to you. You do so much for your team, let them show you the same."

It was then time to tell my team that their leader, whom they probably thought was strong and didn't need to lean on anyone, was about to hand over the reins to take a break and ask them for their prayers for a miracle. I was glad the meeting with them was over the phone. I couldn't look them in the eyes while telling them this news; no one needed to see me cry at work. My team is my "work family" and when one of us is down the entire team jumps in and provides support. It was no different with me. I felt the love and support immediately and throughout the entire journey.

I called my holistic doctor, with whom I had been working for years to treat my autoimmune disorder, and told her of my diagnosis. She was so understanding and loving, but not surprised. I have an autoimmune disorder that had not been treated for many years. She had tried to help me but I only listened half of the time to her recommendations. I promised her that after surgery I would come back and do each and every single thing she had been recommending. I was in the "big leagues" now dealing with breast cancer. I needed a healthy immune system to fight any other "invaders" that tried to come in after my cancer was removed.

Key Message: Expand your tribe when you are ready. You will need their support and prayers.

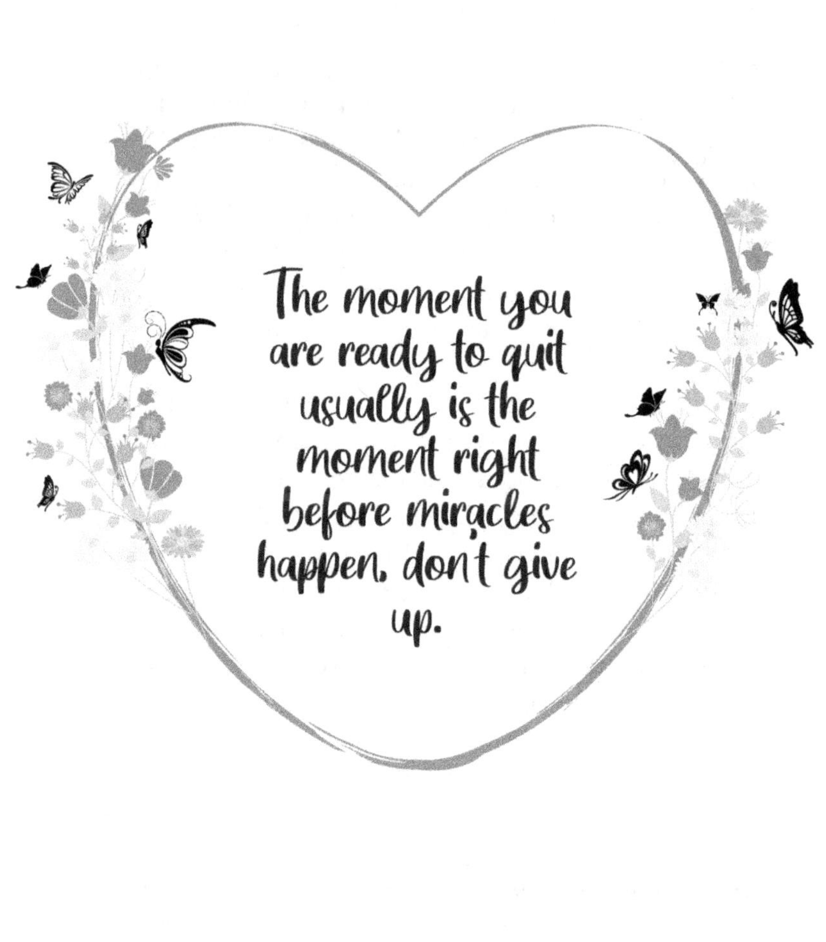
The moment you
are ready to quit
usually is the
moment right
before miracles
happen, don't give
up.

Chapter 6: My miracle(s)

March 13, 2019, 7 am was the date and time for my surgery. Although I could not sleep the night before, I was strangely at peace as I drove to the hospital with my husband. I was in full peace knowing that I had the best surgeons, prayers and a loving family and friends who would be there to care for me when I woke up. The plan was to remove three lymph nodes from around my armpit, to remove the cancer tumor and to have both breasts reduced from a size E to perfect a size C. I don't remember anything about the surgery, just my plastic surgeon's huge smile as he used a cold sharpie to draw on my breasts. I smiled back, thinking of his boob contest comment when I'd first met him. I then fell into a deep sleep and woke up to my husband's warm smile. After surgery I stayed in the hospital for only a few hours and was then sent home to recover. Was the surgery painful? No. But the post-operation period was. I had nothing to compare this surgery to except childbirth, and this pain was much worse than that. But I really I didn't care about the pain. I had woken up and I was alive. My cancer tumor was removed and I was told that cancer had not spread to the lymph nodes under my left armpit—praise God! When my breast surgeon called my husband later, she said I had several lymph nodes within my breast tissue, which is highly unusual. The nodes were covering my tumor and she had been fearful that the cancer cells might have spread to those nodes that had made a "nest" around the tumor. But she said those nodes were also clear. Another miracle for me!

After three days, it was time for us to go back to my surgeon's office to have my drainage tubes and surgery site looked at. I was in pain but I was excited to see her and thank her. When she walked into the room she had a huge smile on her face. She said I looked good and the surgery had gone very well. She then said the pathology results had come back and. . . . my cancer was NOT triple negative after all! I cried, my husband cried—these were tears of pure joy and gratefulness for another miracle. To top off the great news, she said because the estrogen in my tumor was very low I would not need to take an estrogen blocker, which can make women very ill. Praise God! I never told my surgeon about my prayers, my family and friend's prayers. The first person I called was my mom and best friend. "Your prayers worked!" I screamed. "My cancer is *not* triple negative and all my margins are clear." That night I slept for hours, in peace, knowing God answers prayers and does provide healing miracles.

My daughter stayed with me after my surgery. She knew the surgery was a huge success, with no lymph nodes involved, and I finally told her that I'd received a miracle, that the original diagnosis was wrong. I was happy I had waited to tell her until after the final pathology was done and the skilled doctors could see the tumor for an accurate reading. Had I told her earlier she would have used Dr. Google like I had and been worried sick needlessly.

> *Key message: Until you have your cancer tumor removed and examined along with the lymph nodes, it is difficult to know the exact makeup of your cancer and you cannot start to formulate your treatment plan. The initial biopsy is not always accurate!*

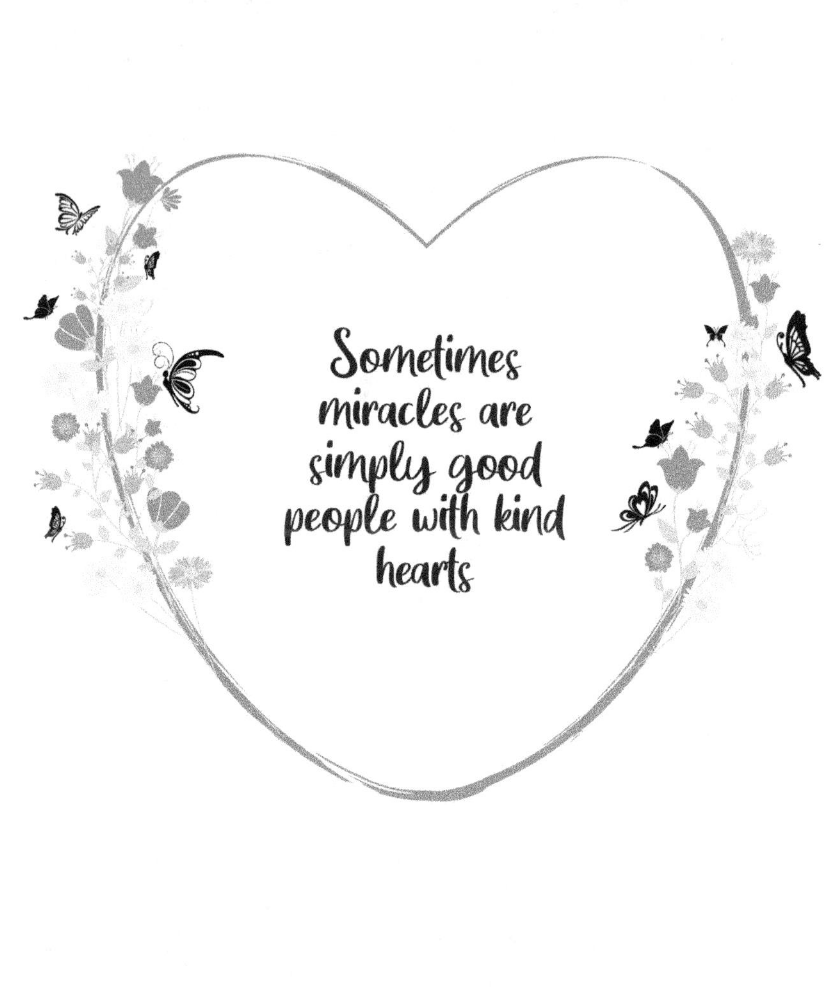
Sometimes
miracles are
simply good
people with kind
hearts

Chapter 7: It is not over until the bell has rung!

After you hear the words "You have cancer" it's a huge relief to have the tumor surgically removed. .You believe that it is gone and now you can heal. For me, I needed to surround myself with a tribe of experts, family and friends to get me through the next phase of my journey. I had to heal and I didn't realize that I would not be able to do as many things during the healing process as I had hoped. I needed to rest. My body forced me to rest and that is exactly what I needed in order to heal.

I had read so many uplifting books about how the body and mind can heal themselves. I was hopeful and knew that God would be with me every step of the way. In fact, I asked for messages on where to go next, and He answered them. If for some reason I didn't understand the message the first time, He sent it again. I thank God that He didn't give up, He just kept sending me the messages.

My surgeon recommended that I meet with an expert radiologist and a medical oncologist regarding my next steps. It was my choice to meet with them; I could have walked away with only having removed the tumor and then started on my healing journey naturally and holistically. Remember, I was at one of the best teaching hospitals in northern California. I had done my research to find the best radiology team in my area and they were at that teaching hospital. I wasn't going to get a second opinion with so many stellar reviews on this hospital and their state-of-the-art radiology equipment. In fact, many folks fly in from other states to use their equipment and I was blessed that it was only a 20-minute drive from my house.

Prior to meeting the radiology team, my husband and I made a pact. We agreed that before we took on any next steps the odds needed to be in our favor. We knew the side effects would take a toll on my body based on my already compromised immune system, and any further treatments needed to have impressive results. We both agreed that the odds needed to be at least 30% favorable or we would decline the treatments and move on to natural remedies. I met the head of the radiology department, a lovely lady who was skilled, knowledgeable and compassionate, who told me that although my tumor was relatively small and was caught early, I would benefit from radiation treatments. In fact, the statistics—and she had plenty of statistics—said that radiation could drop the recurrence of cancer in the same breast by 40%. That was all we needed to hear. It was above the 30% my husband and I had agreed on so I was in—sign me up! I was told that I needed radiation treatments every day for four weeks, and then we could talk about a "boost" in the fifth week. I left there feeling good that in four to five weeks this step to healing would be behind me.

> *Key message: Know your odds and listen to your gut!*

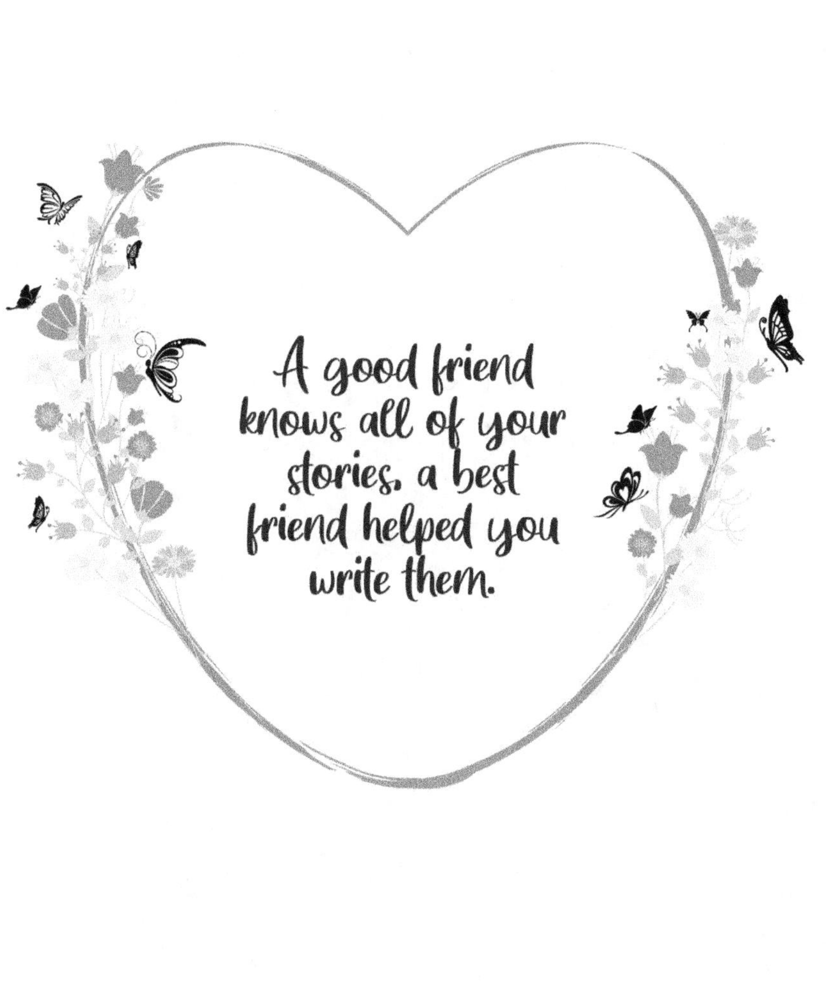
A good friend
knows all of your
stories, a best
friend helped you
write them.

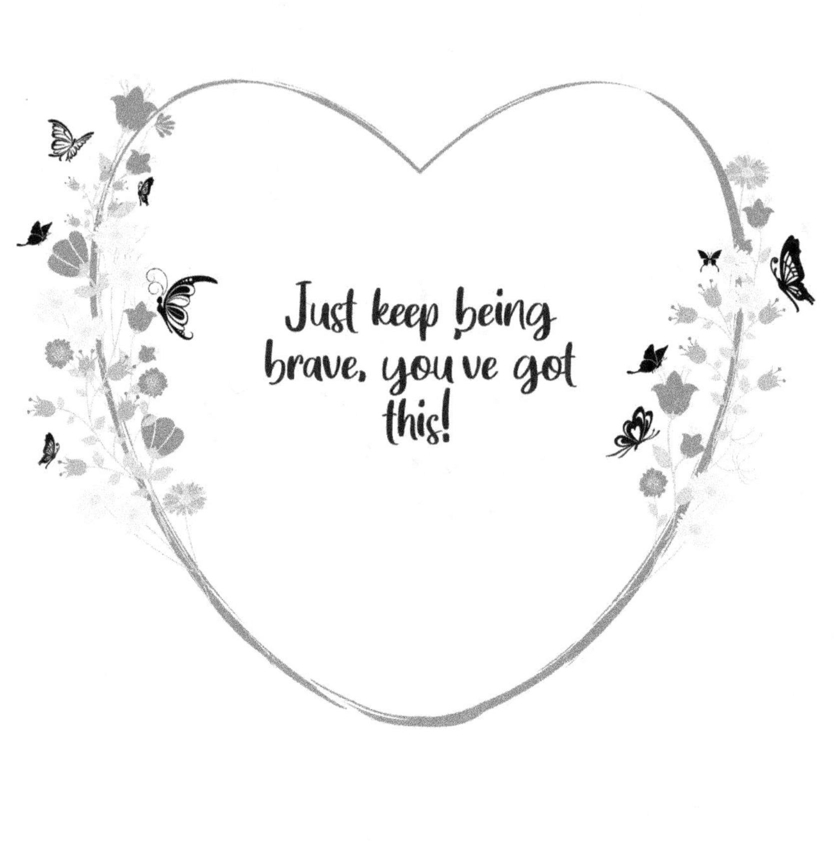
Just keep being
brave, you've got
this!

Chapter 8: The other C word

Unfortunately there are a couple of other C words I used during my journey that I am not proud of. But this is my story and I am sharing it unfiltered.

The radiology team said that it is protocol to also meet with a medical oncologist, otherwise known as the "chemo doctor." I have to admit hearing her say the other C word, chemo, scared me. I had read hundreds of articles about the damaging effects that chemotherapy has on the immune system. I didn't think I was going to have chemo treatments based on the stage of my cancer—the effects simply weren't worth it and I'd read that chemotherapy has a success rate of only 2–3%. In addition, my trusted holistic doctor who was treating my autoimmune disorder strongly suggested I should not place foreign chemicals into my body. She was also not thrilled that I'd opted for radiation. I prayed on this. I should have listened to God and not gone for a consultation. It had to be by far one of the worst experiences during my healing journey.

Not only did I torture myself by going to one medical oncologist, I went to two. Not sure what I was thinking—clearly I wasn't. I had a message from God saying not to do chemo. I kept seeing the same 2–3% statistics over and over. Both chemo doctors said the same thing; they both agreed they over-treat 85% percent of their patients, meaning over 85 people out of 100 did not need chemo or it did nothing for them—what the heck?

The common side effects that both doctors explained to me where horrific, and with my autoimmune system, they would be even worse. When I explained to one of them that, based on what I was hearing, I would not be using chemo but rather radiation only, she had the nerve to say, "Do you want to die?" Through her evil smile while saying those words I saw the devil. God showed me His true colors and showed me the face of the devil. I was so angry that I grabbed my jacket, accidently leaving my purse in the room, which my poor husband grabbed on the way out as I screamed in my loudest voice, "YOU ARE NOT GOD. DON'T EVER TELL SOME-ONE THEY MIGHT DIE. YOU ARE THE DEVIL AND A C__T." I used the other C word, which is only reserved for the worst of the worst—the C word I don't like to use. I know my actions were not "God-like." They were rude and obnoxious and I am not proud of them. I asked God for forgiveness.

Two weeks later that oncologist even had the nerve to send me a $500 bill for her time, even though I'd walked out. Needless to say the bill was sent back—without a check but including another not-so-nice note. I have a temper—not one of my best qualities, and something I am trying to change. I did pray for her and all of the other patients who would see her next, that she watches her words more carefully and that her patients make the best decision for *them* and not based on her scare tactics.

Key Message: Listen to your gut and heart. This is *your body and mind. God is our healer.*

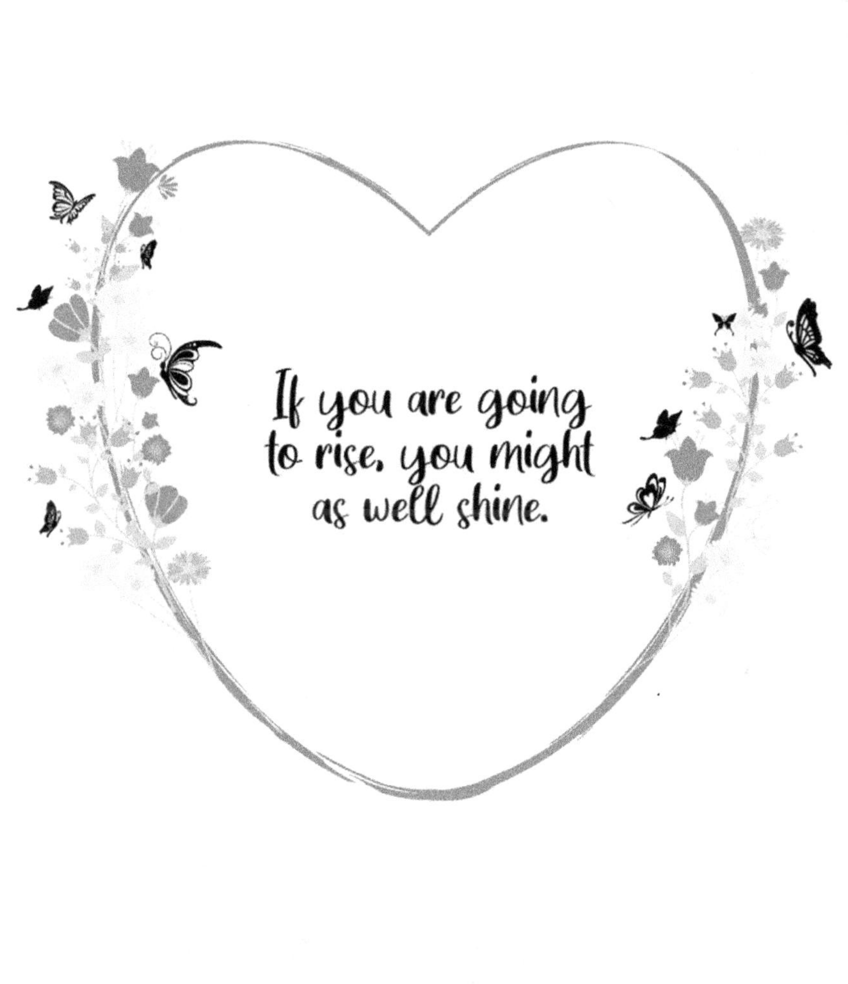
If you are going
to rise, you might
as well shine.

Chapter 9: What do snowflakes, lipstick and gangsta rap have in common?

Before I was allowed to begin my daily radiation treatments, my surgery scars had to heal. I also needed to be able to lift my left arm above my head. This took 30 days of physical therapy and rest. I was able to enjoy Easter break with my family in Scottsdale, Arizona. My mom met us there. This was the first time I saw her after telling her the news over the phone. She'd begged to come out while I was recovering but I didn't want her there watching me sleep. I wanted her with me when I could visit and have her motivate me for what would come next. We had such an amazing week of day trips, floating in the pool and laughing. My daughter was there too, which was icing on the cake. The day after we left Arizona, my treatments began.

I started on a Monday. I asked that my appointment time be early on the first day. I was able to choose the time and I wanted to beat traffic. I wanted these treatments over early so I could see my holistic doctor for treatments after my radiation.

My husband came to the first treatment with me. They had already made a mold of my upper body so that the radiation machine would only target the radiation to the tumor area and surrounding tissue versus impacting my heart or lungs. The hospital had sent a video of the machine and procedure so I knew what to expect. What I didn't expect was how kind, funny and loving the radiation team was. The procedure took less than 15 minutes. My husband was shocked to see me come out dressed so quickly. I told him that it was a breeze and I would be driving myself to the rest of the treatments so he could work. He was not having that. He felt that I needed a driver and he would be it. Guess who won that argument? I did. The next day I drove myself and the hospital even had valet parking. I got the royal treatment. Who needed a driver? Not me!

A beautiful young blond girl was assigned as my technician for the remainder of my four weeks of treatment. She said the hospital usually played the patient's favorite music while they were getting treatments. She asked what she could play to relax me. I know she was thinking this 50+-year-old mom would ask for elevator piano music. But when I said 1990s Gangsta Rap Volume 10 she burst out laughing. When I proceeded to name the artists she knew I was serious. From the moment she blasted the first rap song and she and I sang the lyrics, we were bonded.

She also said it helps to visualize healing during these treatments. What worked for me was visualizing beautiful white snowflakes as my cells—clean, white, sparkly cells that were healthy and working great to boost my immune system. White snowflakes will always have a special place in my heart as a result.

Anyone who says radiation doesn't hurt isn't telling the truth. The procedure itself didn't hurt. However, by the fourth day of the treatment my skin was raw, swollen, itchy and red. You can only imagine what it is like on day 20 and 25. Ouch! I had zero luck with the creams, potions and lotions suggested by the radiology department. What worked for me was pure aloe gel, Lindi Skin Cooler Rolls, essential oils and continuing to use the heart pillows I'd had since surgery under my armpits for support.

Each day I went to radiation I tried to look my best. I didn't want to look sick and tired. I wanted to get back to normal, and normal for me is doing my make-up and hair and getting dressed in my best. I was swollen, tired and in pain but I remember what my southern aunts and grandma told me: "Don't leave home without your lips on." They would be proud. I never did not leave home "without my lips on" and my beautiful technician said each day, "I see you have your shiniest lip gloss on again."

With the gangsta rap playing, visualizing clean, white snowflakes flowing through my body and wearing my pink lip-gloss I made it. After four weeks of daily treatments and with a swollen, red and raw breast, I rang the bell! That part of my healing journey was now behind me.

I should mention that the hospital did not perform the last week of the boost. They said that it would only possibly help an additional 2%. Remember that pact I'd made with my husband about 30%—well you can see why I wasn't going to place more radiation in my body. In fact, the head of the radiation team agreed with my position on this, as did as my holistic immune doctor.

> *Key message: Do what makes you smile during your treatments—music heals!*

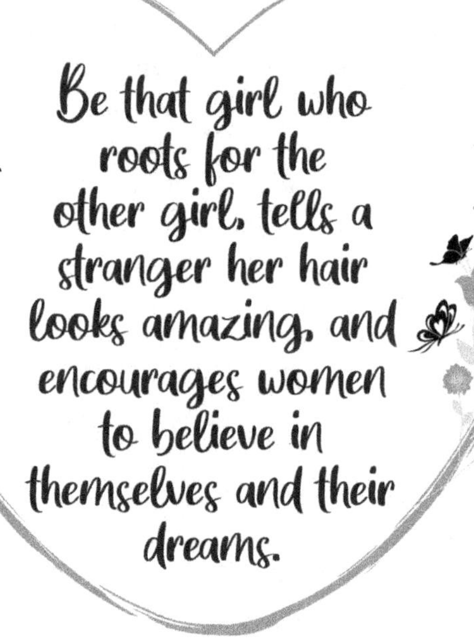

Be that girl who
roots for the
other girl, tells a
stranger her hair
looks amazing, and
encourages women
to believe in
themselves and their
dreams.

Chapter 10: Radiation and IV buddies

I was getting radiation treatments at the same time every weekday for four weeks. I had my morning routine. I chose to drive myself and I truly needed the quiet time to pray and reflect on the day. I had my green tea in hand. Highway 280 in the San Francisco Bay area is very beautiful in the morning with less traffic than some alternatives, so that was the route I chose. The hospital had valet parking and I got to know the parking attendants fairly well by my last appointment. During my early morning appointments I started to see the same faces in the waiting room. We all knew why we were there: for radiation treatments. But no one talked about the reason. There was a young woman to whom I decided to introduce myself. She too was going to have the same treatments as me for four weeks on her left breast. After our introduction, we bonded with our stories of how and when we were diagnosed. As the days went on, our stories turned to how we were treating our sore, red, swollen and itchy breasts. We both agreed that we were on our own to figure out how to get relief—everything that was recommend by the doctor didn't work. Thank goodness for Amazon reviews. We both found relief by trial and error and each of us found the concoction that worked, at least temporarily, so we could sleep through the night. The only thing that really works is stopping radiation to let your body heal. I have to say that the pain become worse two weeks after my treatments ended. I was not expecting that at all. However, the doctors explained that it's the cumulative effect of the treatments.

My radiation buddy and I still text each other to see how the other is feeling. Although I would not wish cancer or radiation on anyone, it was so nice to see the same warm smile each morning and to count down the days until we could ring the bell, get our certificate and pin and never look back.

During my radiation treatments, my holistic doctor did everything in her power to ensure that the radiation would not have a negative impact on my already compromised Immune system. She recommended that for the duration of my radiation treatments I should receive a high dose of vitamin C—75,000 mg via IV—and ozone therapy to clean my blood twice a week. I was beyond blessed that at the time of my treatments, my holistic doctor and the IV treatments were less than two miles from my home.

Although I was starting to get tired from the radiation treatments, the vitamin C and ozone IVs gave me so much energy. I felt like the poison I was getting in the morning from the radiation was flushed out of my system by those amazing IVs. I can only pray that that was the case. In my heart I believe these treatment were successful. I felt great and my scars from the surgery were healing better than expected because of these treatments. But none of these treatments were covered by insurance. It was very expensive and I was fortunate to be able to get them.

At the IV center the appointments lasted between four and six hours. I was in the room with the most loving and supporting patients who were trying to heal from various illnesses: Hashimoto's Disease, Lyme disease, cancer and more. I so looked forward to seeing my IV buddies twice a week and sharing stories—not doom and gloom stories, but stories of hope and divine health. Unfortunately, the IV center close to my home closed and my IV buddies had to find other centers. However, we stay in contact with each other, checking in and providing each other healing words of encouragement. There was one special lady who I knew wasn't feeling well. Each day, however, her smile lit up the room, her skin radiating beauty. She reminded me so much of my beautiful grandmother who was dear to me. When choosing my IV chair I would park myself close to her so I could feel her positive radiant energy, hoping some would rub off on me.

I am blessed beyond measure to have found such a supportive and loving group of people who were strangers when I walked in, not knowing what to expect. God brings special people into our lives for a reason and I know He brought my IV buddies into mine when I needed them the most.

Key Message: Smile at strangers; you may make a friend. Rest, rest, rest during radiation. Care for your skin a few times a day. Be sure the lotions and potions you use on your breast are organic and non-toxic.

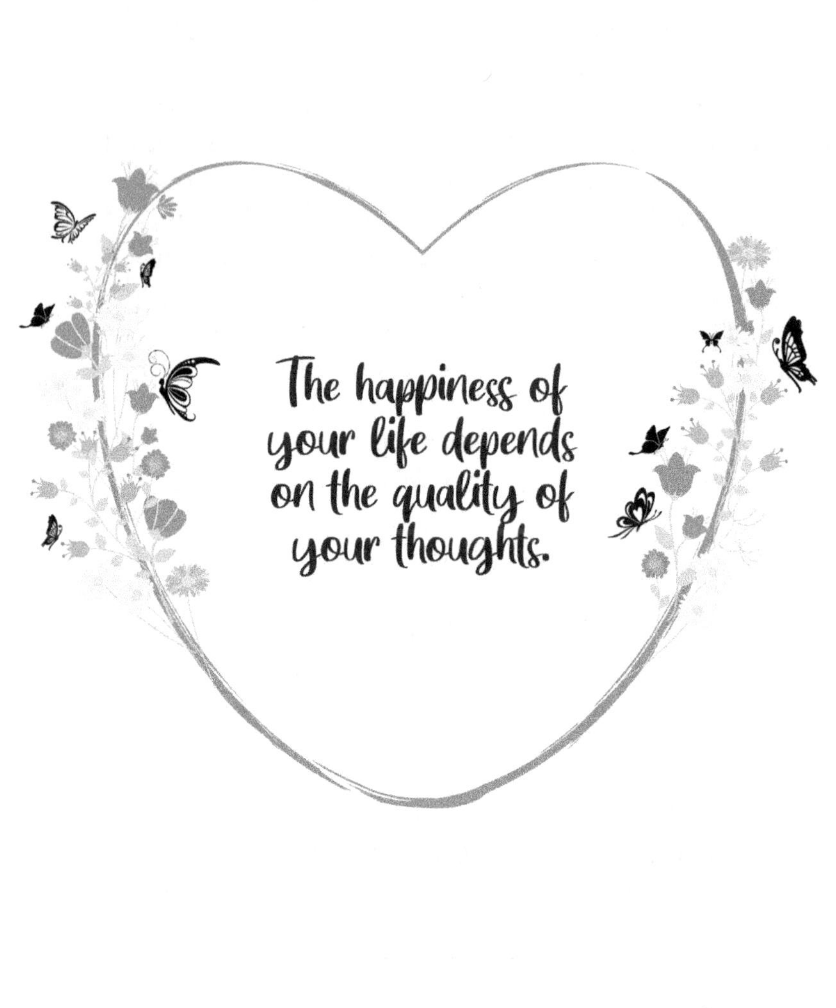

The happiness of
your life depends
on the quality of
your thoughts.

Chapter 11: Healed in Topanga

*N*ow that the cancer tumor was removed and my radiation treatments were behind me, I knew I needed to heal my mind and thoughts. My daughter asked that I watch a documentary called *Heal*. How did my 24-year-old daughter, who is healthy, recommend this film to me? I believe in my heart it was another message from God. I now listen and act versus questioning the message.

Heal features Dianne Porchia for her healing work with advanced stage cancer clients who remain cancer-free four years after diagnosis with stage IV cancer. Dianne's unique holistic approach to healing integrates the principles and practice of mind-body medicine and a spiritual perspective that supports optimum immune function through high-stress life challenges.

After watching this film, I was so inspired and was hoping to read more books on the topic of releasing emotions. I turned to my husband and said, "I wish I knew where Topanga was. I would do anything to meet Dianne." I thought Topanga was in another country. Little did I know that Topanga was only five hours from my home. My next thought was, "Is Dianne famous due to this film and likely retired?" I reached out to Dianne's assistant and was able to book three days with her in her home in Topanga Canyon in Los Angeles. The only time Dianne had available was in early June, which could not have been more perfect for me since we needed to move my son home for summer college break two days after my Topanga healing, and his college was on the drive home. Divine timing at its best! I learned so much from Dianne, however, what was key to my healing was her healing methods to integrate effective stress reduction techniques, mind-body medicine principles and body-mind-heart-soul wellness practices into my daily routine for creating life in balance. She trained me that wellness means looking at the five levels of my life:

- **Physical Level:** Diet, nutrition, exercise, work habits and lifestyle factors.
- **Mental Level:** Thoughts, beliefs and values motivate behaviors, which are either supportive or not supportive of one's goals.
- **Emotional Level:** Feelings and emotions follow thoughts, beliefs and values and affect the physical body on a cellular level.
- **Subconscious Level:** Thoughts and feelings hidden from the conscious mind that motivate behavior and can feed unhealthy thoughts
- **Spiritual Level:** Source of spiritual growth, personal healing, love, forgiveness, compassion. The heart and soul level is where all healing takes place.

Dianne told me to write this message down and look at it every time I had to make a decision: ***"What is the most Self-loving, Self-nurturing and Self-honoring choice I can make in this moment?"***

I will not go into detail on what was discussed over my three days with Dianne; these were private things I have shared with only a few. I will say that those were the best three days of healing on an emotional level I have ever experienced. Dianne was able to dig deep and find the reason why I was a perfectionist and why good is never good enough, why I thought I was responsible for everyone's happiness and looked for approval versus practicing self-care when I knew I had a faulty immune system. I will be forever grateful for the time I spent with Dianne in the beautiful Topanga Canyon. When I think of someone who is at total peace with themselves, I think of Dianne. I will continue to look to her as a role model for creating holistic health and balance. My husband says to think of Dianne as your NORTH STAR.

> *Key Message: You must clear your toxic emotions before you can fully heal.*

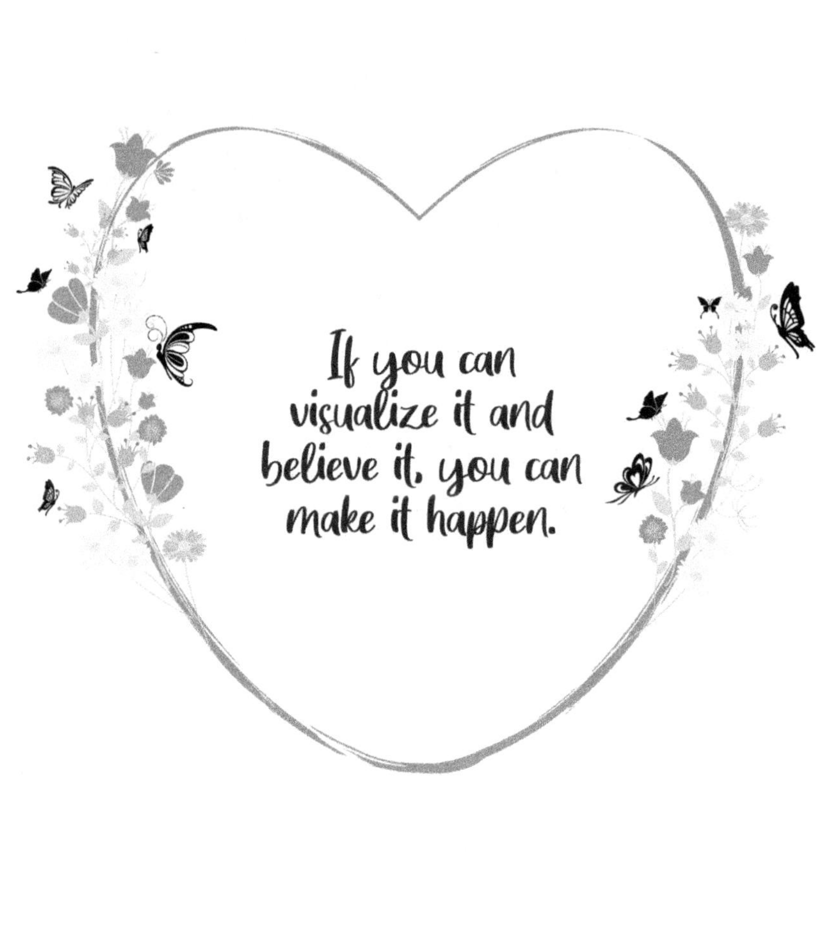
If you can
visualize it and
believe it, you can
make it happen.

Chapter 12: More messages, prayers and healing touch

My car license plate that I have had for many years reads 2Belev. Many people have asked me what it means and I respond, "I believe in miracles. I believe anything is possible. I believe in myself and I believe in God." I now believe you should do whatever is in your power and your belief system to fight for divine health. There are many things that I pursued while searching for spiritual ways in which to heal. Although cancer is out of my body, I need all of the good energy, angels and God to keep me healthy and to forever heal my immune system to detect issues and fight.

Here are a few of my healing experiences:

Reiki

I adore my Reiki master. My first experience with her (before cancer) was amazing. I immediately felt a change in my wellbeing, and once I had the cancer diagnosis she was one of the first persons I called to provide peace over my emotions. My Reiki master uses a technique of light touch and above-the-body energy sweeping, which is calming or grounding.

Laying of hands

One of my healers who has helped me with manual lymphatic massages invited me to San Francisco to meet a wonderful healer who will lay hands on a person and send a message from God. She knew I was open to anything and everything that would give me peace and healing. I told my husband of the plan and he was excited as his mother had asked her priest to lay hands on her when she went through breast cancer.

The day came for me to meet my friend, who was also bringing someone who needed healing. Thank GOD my husband joined me because I needed a witness of what was to happen that night. We walked into a home full of loving Christians. I knew no one, but it didn't matter. I knew I was sent there for another healing message. I felt loved. The healer asked that anyone who needed a special healing meet her in the living room. I went straight to the living room and waited my turn. I saw her lay hands on the sick and many dropped to the floor crying. I thought to myself, "What if I don't drop to the ground, am I still being healed?" Now I was nervous.

The healer walked to me and asked me why I was there. I told her that I was healing from breast cancer and needed it to be healed forever. She laid her hands on my left breast. I'd never told her which breast had the cancer, by the way. She said words to God that only she understood. After she was finished, she looked at me and said, "You are the fortieth person who will receive a special healing from God." She said number 40 is a special number and is mentioned several times in the Bible. She said, "You are a leader and many people listen to you" (I'm not sure that is correct). She also said, "Please tell your story." I said to her that "is a promise I already made to God." She smiled, and we both cried. If my husband hadn't been there to witness this with me no one would believe me. I will never forget that night in that small, warm and loving San Francisco home, which provided another message of love, peace and healing. I am number 40 and so proud of it!

Apparition Hill, Medjugorje, Bosnia and Herzegovina

We had a family summer trip planned to Croatia at the end of June. We'd planned and paid for this trip long before my diagnosis and having this amazing trip to look forward to was always in my mind while I was healing. After my experience in San Francisco with the healer my husband decided to book a side trip to Bosnia to visit the town of Medjugorje. Worshippers pray around the statue of the Virgin Mary on top of Apparition Hill outside the holy site of Medjugorje, in the country of Bosnia and Herzegovina. Countless pilgrims have gone there seeking physical and spiritual healing. This was about a four-hour ride each way from where we were staying in Croatia. When we arrived at the spot I could immediately feel that this was a very holy place of peace and love. It was a warm day and the hike up a steep hill filled with large rocks was difficult to traverse. I am so grateful my family agreed to go to the top with me. I wanted them all there, praying for more healing and thanking God for the miracles already given. I will never forget that day and even now when I am having a hard day, I think of the statue, the warmth and peace I felt.

The following bible verses helped me focus on my healing and gave me peace:

- I can do all things through Christ which strengtheneth me. Philippians 4:13
- I shall not die, but live and declare the works of the Lord. PSALM 118:17
- He sent His word and healed them, and delivered them from their destructions. PSALM 107:20
- Be strong and courageous, do not be afraid or discouraged, for the Lord will personally go ahead of you. He will be with you; he will neither fail you nor abandon you. Deuteronomy 31:7,8
- By his stripes I was healed. Isaiah 53:5
- God hath not given us sprit of fear; but power and love, and of a sound mind. 2 Timothy 1:7
- Therefore I say to you, whatever things you ask when you pray, believe that you will receive them, and you will have them. Mark 11:24
- And these signs shall follow those who believe, they will lay hands on the sick and they will recover. Mark 16:17–18

Key Message: Find your spiritual healers and pray!

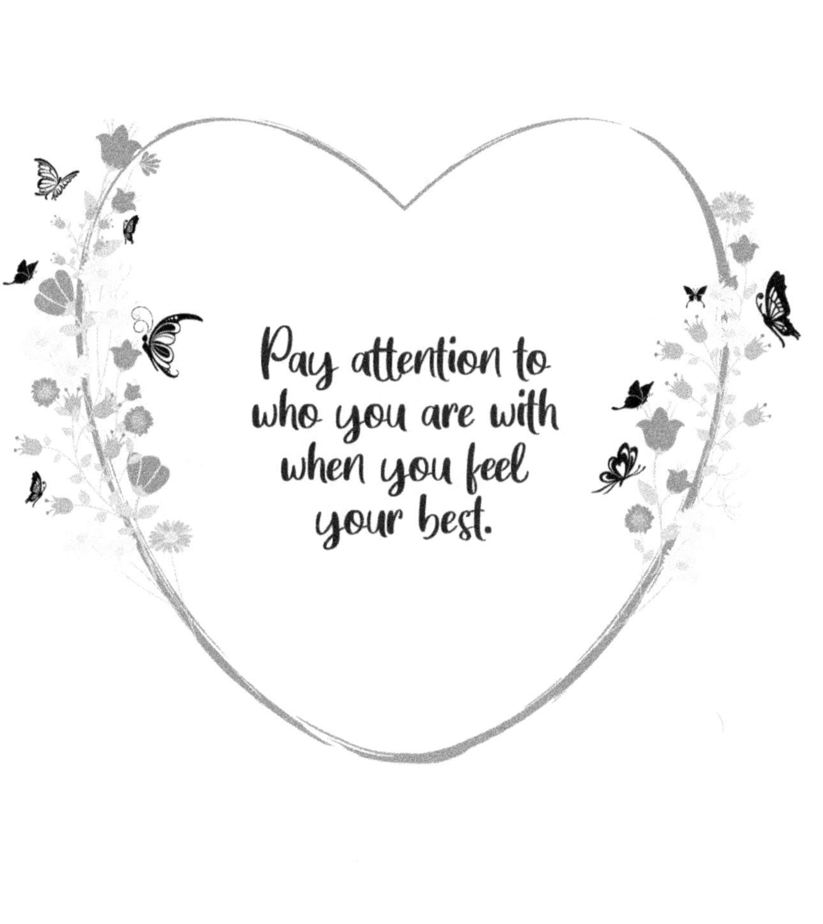

Pay attention to
who you are with
when you feel
your best.

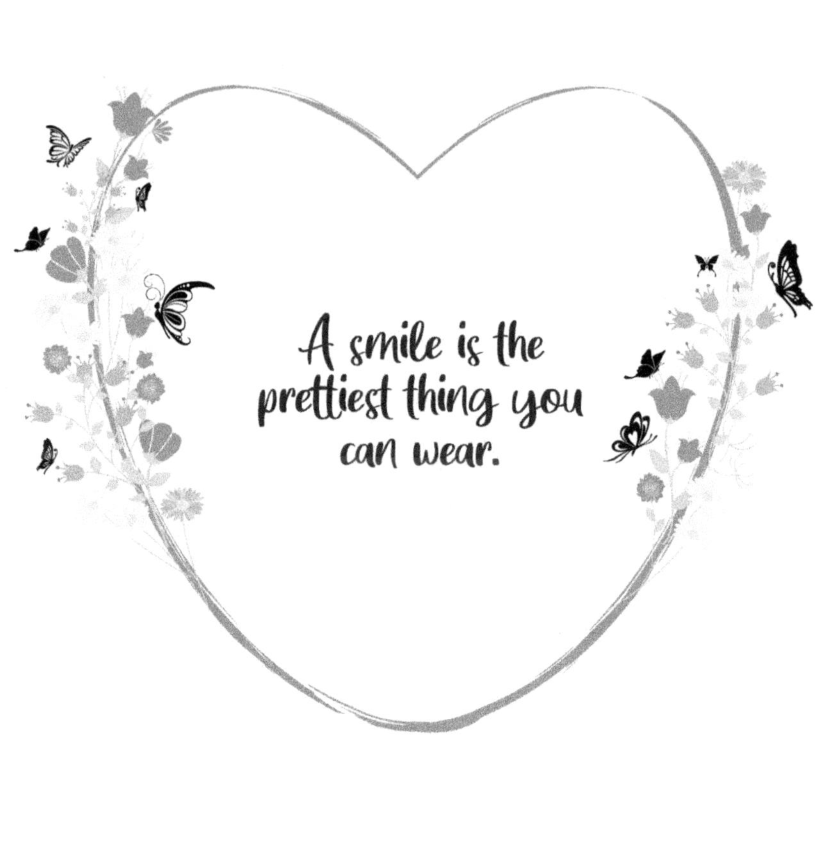
A smile is the
prettiest thing you
can wear.

Chapter 13: My mama always said watch your mouth!

My holistic team was surprised to hear that I still had four "silver" fillings containing metals that were releasing toxins into my body, overwhelming my already compromised immune system. I wasn't sure if it would really make a difference if I removed my fillings, but what was shocking is that the four teeth that had the metal in them tied directly to the breast meridian according to Chinese medicine. That scared me so much that I immediately made an appointment with a biological dentist who removed them using the SMART method (Safe Mercury Amalgam Removal Technique). There are very few dentists who perform this safe method of metal filling removal and I was grateful I had one about an hour away from me. He told me that my fillings were made of mercury and that vapors are released each time you chew or have a warm drink. In essence, I'd had these fillings for over 25 years and had been poisoning myself.

Oil pulling is something I did before my diagnosis. Oil pulling is an ancient practice that involves swishing oil (I use organic coconut oil) in your mouth to remove bacteria and promote oral hygiene.

I found that oil pulling can kill bacteria in the mouth and improve dental health. Oil pulling is easy to do and involves just a few simple steps:

1. Measure one tablespoon of oil, such as coconut, sesame or olive oil.
2. Swish it around in your mouth for 15–20 minutes, being careful not to swallow any.
3. Spit the oil into a trash can once you're done. Avoid spitting it into the sink or toilet, as this can cause a buildup of oil, which may lead to clogging.
4. Rinse your mouth well using water before eating or drinking anything.

Repeat these steps a few times per week, or up to three times daily. You may also want to work your way up, starting with swishing for just 5 minutes and increasing the duration until you're able to do it for a full 15–20 minutes.

> *Key Message: Find a holistic dentist to remove your mercury fillings with the SMART method.*

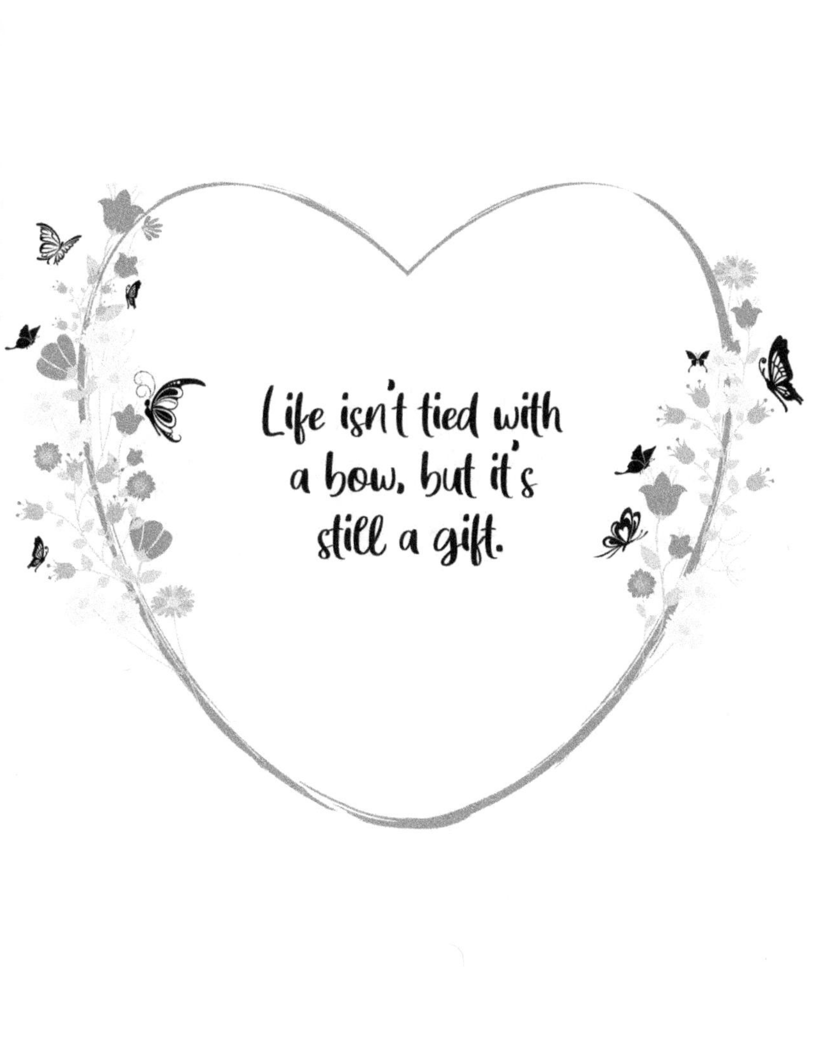

Life isn't tied with
a bow, but it's
still a gift.

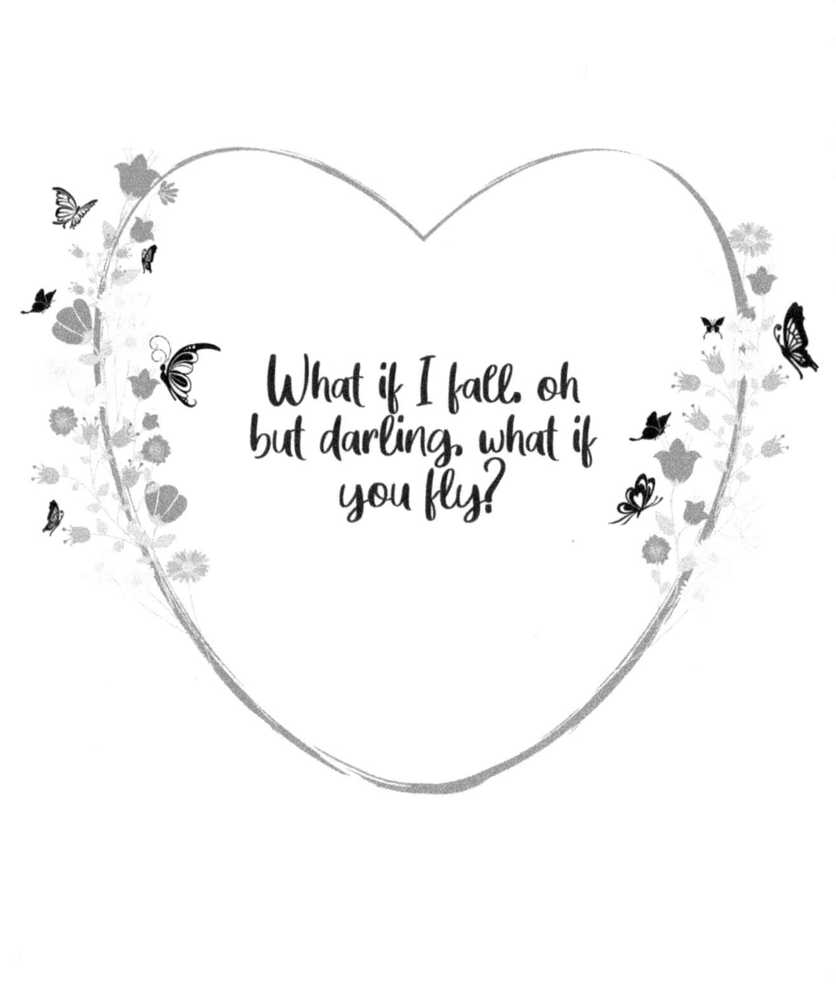

What if I fall, oh
but darling, what if
you fly?

Chapter 14: Willing to try anything for divine health

The immune system is ultimately what heals our bodies from diseases like cancer. A healthy immune system is the body's natural protection mechanism. My husband repeats this to me often: "Everyone has cancer cells in their body. Healthy people are not getting cancer—their immune system is able to fight it!"

I have read numerous books and hundreds of articles about having a healthy immune system. Here are some of the holistic things I have used to improve my immune system and that are working for me.

Eat organic—No sugar, alkaline diet and filtered water
Prior to cancer I was eating loads of sugar when I was stressed. I had no idea that sugar feeds cancer so the moment I heard my diagnosis I immediately changed the food I ate and the water I drank to ensure my body was in an alkaline state versus acidic. My alkaline diet was primarily fresh organic vegetables, with little meat and that only grass-fed. I stopped consuming any sugar, dairy, wheat or other high-gluten grains. I test my pH levels every day using pH strips and try to ensure my pH is 7.0 or higher.

Chiropractor

I receive monthly chiropractor adjustments to keep my spine healthy, which then allows my nervous system and immune system to work optimally.

Lymphatic drainage

During my surgery some lymph nodes were removed and my arm and breast felt tight and sore. My lymphatic practitioner believes that the main function of the lymphatic system is detoxification, but it also plays an important role in immunity. Lymphatic drainage is a light massage that gently pushes the toxins out of the lymph nodes and reduces inflammation.

Castor oil packs

My breast was swollen after my radiation treatments, and still is over six months after my last treatment. My holistic doctor recommended castor oil packs to reduce the inflammation, which was helped me greatly. I use castor oil that is cold pressed, without hexane, and is 100% pesticide-free.

Castor Oil Pack Instructions

1. **Prepare 3 layers of cotton flannel.** Fold or cut the cloth into three sheets, creating a pad of adequate size to cover the area to be treated. For example, to use a castor oil pack over the abdominal area, the size of the flannel cloth might be 10"x8" and three sheets thick.

2. **Cut a plastic sheet.** The sheet should be somewhat larger than the flannel cloth. The plastic is used to protect the heating pad from getting oily. Using a plastic garbage bag normally works fairly well,

but it is best to avoid using plastic grocery bags, since they are usually printed with ink on one side, which can dissolve and spread when exposed to castor oil.

3. **Saturate the cloth with castor oil.** Place the flannel cloth on top of the plastic sheet, then saturate it with castor oil. The cloth should be wet, but not dripping. The saturated cloth should then be placed directly on the target area with the plastic sheet on top of it. Your plastic sheet should cover the entire exterior of the saturated flannel, since castor oil is likely to stain any fabric it touches.

4. **Place heating pad over plastic sheet.** Set the heating pad on either a low or medium setting, or higher if it is comfortable. The heat will promote absorption and increase circulation. I keep my pack on for 45 minutes, 3 times a week.

5. **Wash off area.** After using the castor oil pack, cleanse the skin using a washcloth and organic soap. Washing the area helps clear acidic toxins that have been drawn out of the body during the treatment and helps prevent reabsorbing these toxins.

Vitamin C IV therapy

I started receiving high-dose vitamin C IVs (75 grams) during my radiation, and will continue them weekly as long as I can afford them. My holistic doctor believes that, since vitamin C is an anti-oxidant that neutralizes free radicals in the body and stimulates the immune system, it stimulates the production of collagen in cells that improves their cellular stability and helps them resist becoming cancerous.

BioMat

I purchased a BioMat, which uses far infrared light to heat up cells. Most cells are not affected by this heat, but it is claimed that cancer cells are weak and may be killed by this level of heat. Similarly, the theory states that cancer cells favor low body temperature (which means low oxygen levels and high acidity).

Acupuncture

I am blessed to have an on-site acupuncturist at my office. After my weekly treatments I feel calmer, and happier. I have less worry and anxiety and feel more mentally alert and more emotionally stable.

DNA gene testing

We can't do anything about the genes we have but we can change the way they act. When you view your family history and your genes, you know that you will likely head down the same path unless you change the way the genes behave. This can be through very powerful nutritional medicine. I had my genes tested and analyzed by Dr. Kessler and, sure enough, I have problems with detoxification and methylene pathways, which could have contributed to my body being toxic and a host for cancer.

Supplements

These supplements can either be used to prevent cancer developing in the first place or be a part of your protocol if healing from already developed cancer. They all aim to boost the immune system. I recommend working with a holistic doctor to understand what type of supplements work best for you.

My top four supplements are:
- Vitamin D with K
- Curcumin
- Turkey tail mushrooms
- Broccoli sprouts

CBD for pain relief after surgery

After my surgery, which included a reduction of both breasts, I was sore, tender and experienced sharp shooting pains as the nerves were reconnecting. My surgeons prescribed opioids and after two days of taking them with no relief, I reached out to my holistic doctor, who immediately gave me CBD oil capsules. Within hours, I felt relief in my breast as well as my overall wellbeing. I was also advised to use the oil from the capsules to spread directly on my breast, which allowed for even better relief.

THC-FECO oil

I read a very inspirational story of Dee Mani, who cured her triple negative breast cancer with surgery and all-natural remedies, including cannabis in the form of THC-FECO oil. I felt after reading her story I needed to use THC-FECO oil to ensure I remained cancer free.

Epsom salt baths

Salt detox baths are usually made of Epsom salts, which allows the minerals to "draw out" toxins from the body. I believe that soaking in an Epsom salt bath can remove harmful toxins and balance the body. Epsom salts can help detoxify and reduce inflammation while improving mineral and sulfur balance in the body. I personally have used Epsom salts for everything from chronic inflammation to muscle aches to recovering from injuries and pain. I recommend taking an Epson salt bath for at least 20 minutes 3 times a week.

Liquid mind—mindfulness meditation

This is very difficult for me. I am a multi-tasker and worrier by nature, a known fault of mine. When my friends would say I needed to meditate I thought to myself, "How the heck do I clear my mind?" When I tried, my "to-do list" played over and over in my mind. This is when I heard about mindfulness meditation. You're probably familiar with the term meditation, but mindfulness is something many aren't familiar with. When you practice mindfulness you are purposefully filling your mind with something. You are choosing to focus on something. It could be your breathing, a phrase, a body part or an image. The important part is that what you are focusing on is something that is going to help you relax, along with calming your mind and body.

Mindfulness works because it helps you replace your stressful thoughts and anxiety with something positive. If your mind is consumed with anxiety and stress over an upcoming test result, spend some time practicing mindfulness meditation. Purposefully choose something calming to think about. Instead of trying *not* to think about something, purposefully think about something, which is much easier to do.

Essential oils

Essential oils are powerful plant-based chemical compounds that, unlike patented prescription drugs, your body easily absorbs and utilizes. Below are the oils I used during my healing journey.

Frankincense
The king of essential oils, frankincense is revered for its ability to rejuvenate skin when applied topically, to promote cellular health and immunity, and produces a healthy inflammatory response when taken internally, among other benefits. Frankincense is used to support the immune system, fight infection and cure disease and is known as a natural treatment for cancer. The most common benefits are it reduces inflammation, contains cancer-fighting properties and boosts immunity.

Lemon
This oil contains limonene and is very successful with breast cancer. Limonene actually suppresses inflammation, which is the root cause for most diseases.

Lavender
The most important health benefits of lavender include its ability to relieve stress, improve mood, promote restful sleep, lower skin irritation, prevent infections, reduce inflammation, eliminate dandruff and soothe stomach bloating.

Myrrh
This essential oil is well known for its ability to cleanse the mouth and throat. Myrrh also promotes a youthful-looking complexion and offers a soothing sensation to the skin. Try diffusing myrrh oil to promote emotional balance and well-being.

Peppermint
Ancient Egyptians cultivated and used peppermint leaves for indigestion. Peppermint also is frequently used

to reduce inflammation of the mouth or throat. It can help with digestive problems—gas, bloating, nausea, morning sickness and stomach cramps.

Get dirty and grounded . . . it Improves inflammation and immunity

My husband knows that when I say, "Let's go to the beach," even on an overcast day, this means that I want to "ground myself." When I can't get to the beach I take my shoes off while walking my sweet pooch in the grassy park.

My Reiki healer believes that grounding positively affects the inflammatory response and the immune system, and reduces cortisol levels. Grounding is simply removing your shoes and planting your feet on the ground for 5 to 10 minutes.

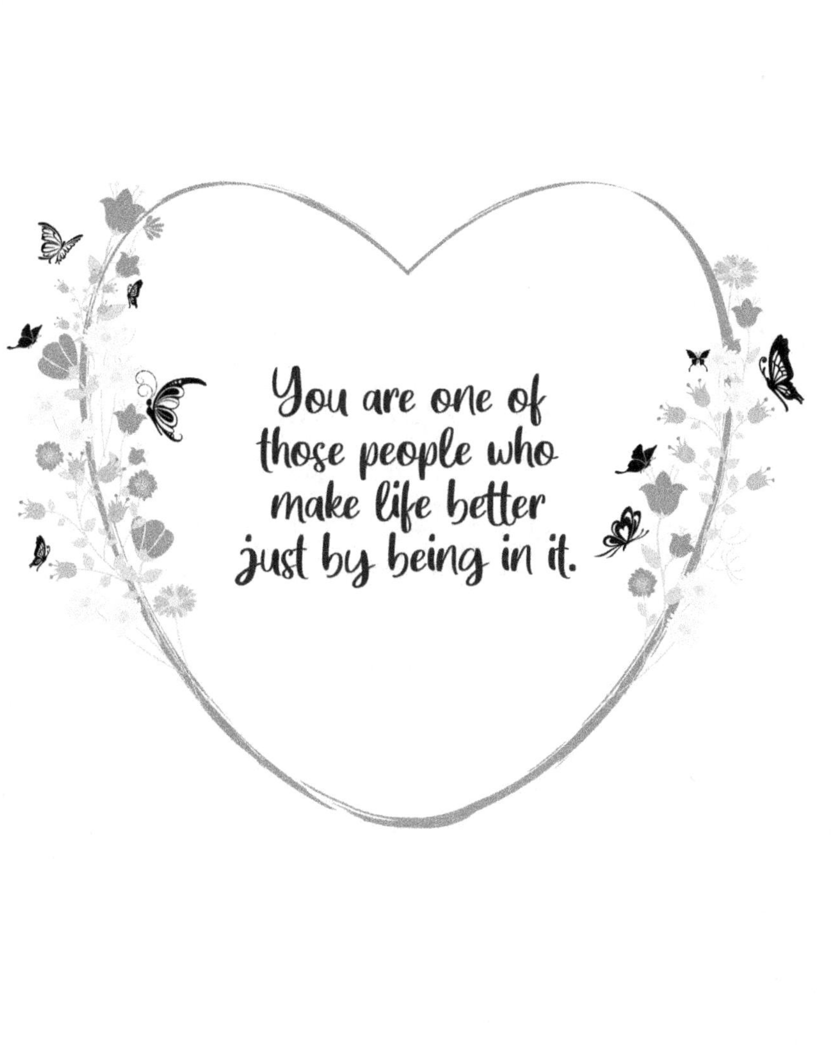
You are one of
those people who
make life better
just by being in it.

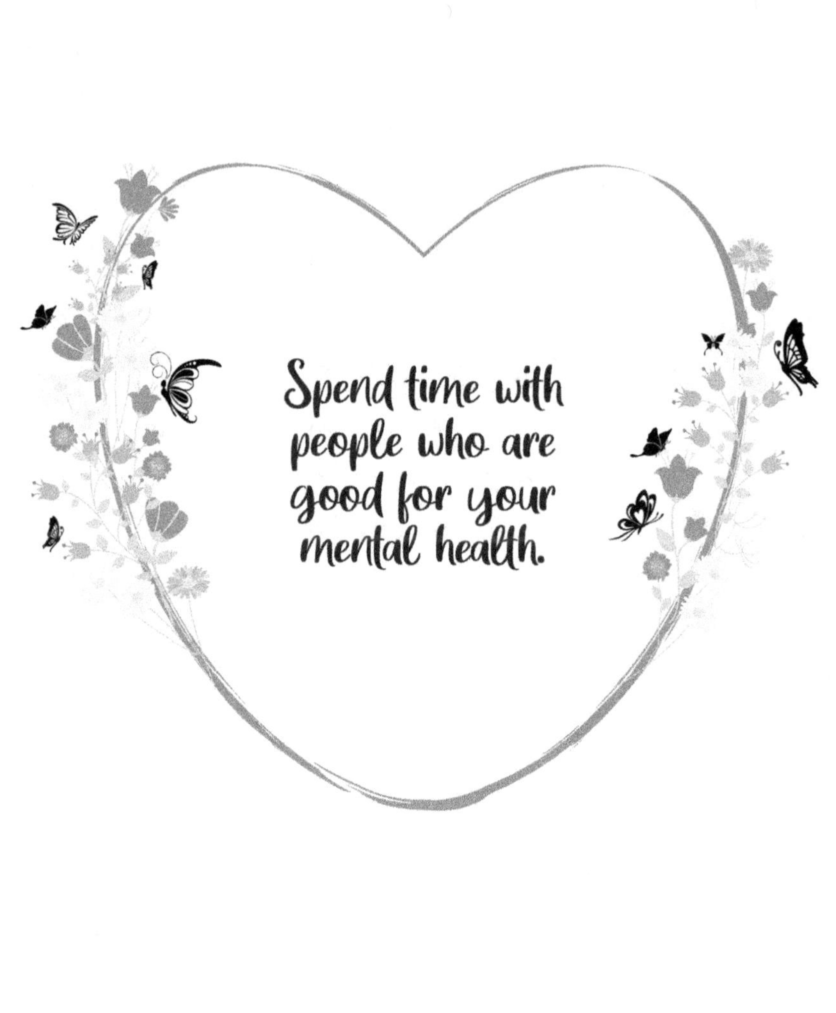

Spend time with
people who are
good for your
mental health.

Chapter 15: Girls love mail and so do I

Many people want to help you when you are sick. I want the same when my friends and loved ones are struggling. During these times one can feel hopelessness.

So when anyone reached out to me asking what they could do I had one simple request. It was simple but meant the world to me. I requested that they send me a card, any card, along with a note of encouragement. These are treasured gems I now hold near and dear to my heart. I keep them all in a special box and look at them from time to time. Going to the mailbox to get mail was one of my simple pleasures during my recovery. All the notes meant the world to me and touched me in ways I will never forget.

One of the letters came from a complete stranger.

It came from on organization called Girls Love Mail. I plan to host an event at my company so that we can show our love to the women who may only receive one letter of encouragement. Please consider writing a letter—you will change someone's day for the better!

The Gift of Hand-Written Letters to Women Newly Diagnosed with Breast Cancer
(from the website girlslovemail.com)

A hand-written letter has the special power to heal. Girls Love Mail collects your hand-written letters of encouragement, bundles them, and sends them, via the caring staff at cancer centers, to women newly diagnosed with breast cancer. Every letter is a gift from you to a woman going through a difficult time.

Anyone can write a letter! All it takes is a little of your time and the cost of a postage stamp to help a woman newly diagnosed with breast cancer.

From the Founder & Author Gina L. Mulligan
Dear Friend,

Letters are sacred mementos we lovingly save in decorative boxes. Yet the gentle beauty of a hand-written letter seems hidden in our age of text messages and emails. After working for five years on a novel comprised entirely of letters, I felt connected to what I consider the lost art of letter writing. However, not until I was diagnosed with breast cancer did I understand that a few words on paper were more than just a keepsake. A hand-written letter is a gift with the ultimate power to heal.

Having just turned 40 and in the throes of writing my novel, being told I had cancer was a shock. But it wasn't the day of my diagnosis that changed my life. The true change came a few weeks later when I started receiving well wishes. I received over 200 letters, mostly from friend of friends. The letters said I was already a hero without telling me I needed to try a special diet or exercise plan.

I was touched by the letters and began wondering if other breast cancer patients were receiving this special form of support. After I won my battle with breast cancer, I knew just what I had to do.

Starting Girls Love Mail was one of those AHA moments. Anyone with a desire to encourage a woman can write a letter. Letter writers of all ages and from across the country are joining us. I hope you will too! All it takes is a little of your time and the cost of a stamp. I know what receiving letters meant to me. I encourage you to give it a try and see how much writing one will mean to you.

Best wishes,
Gina L. Mulligan, Founder

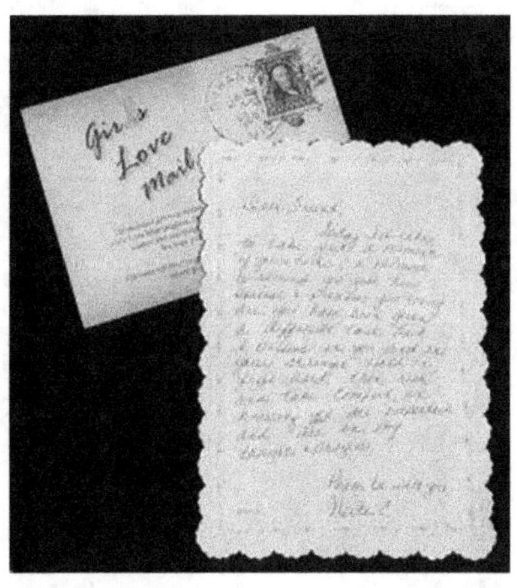

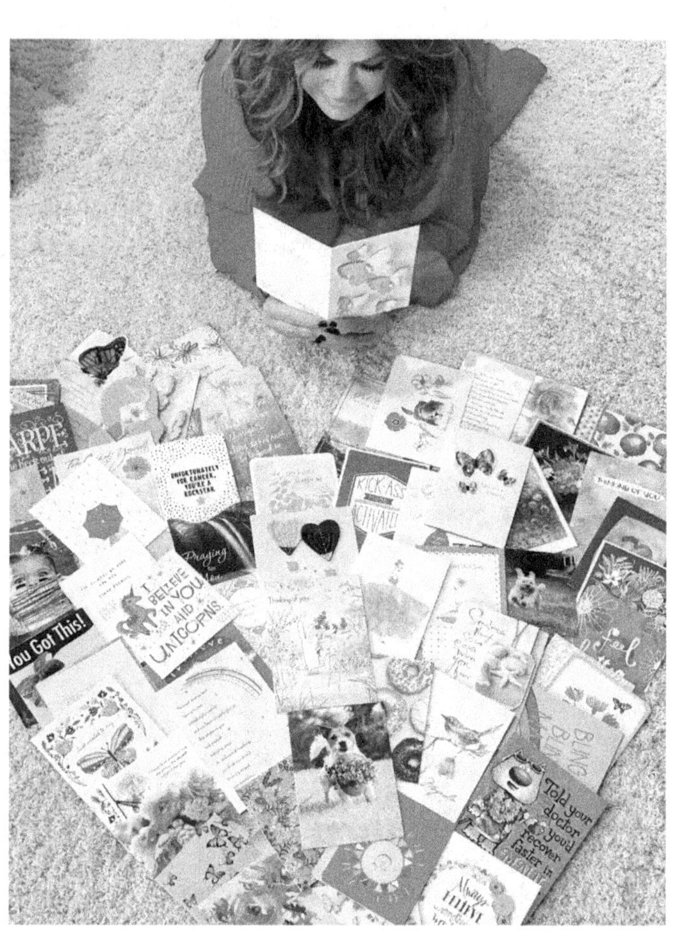

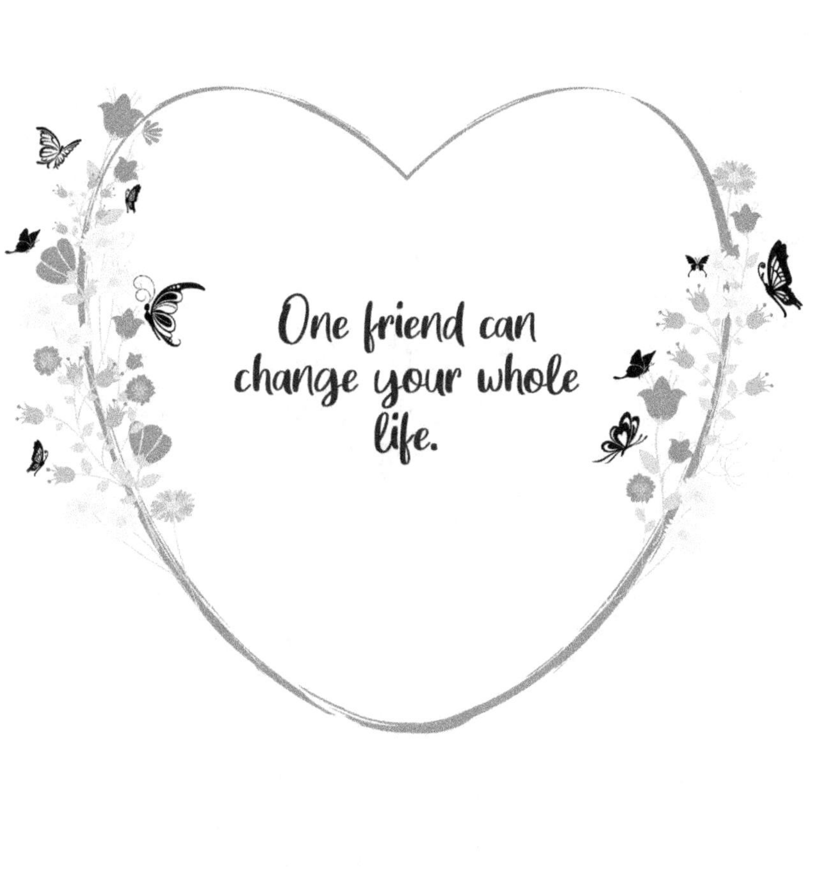
One friend can
change your whole
life.

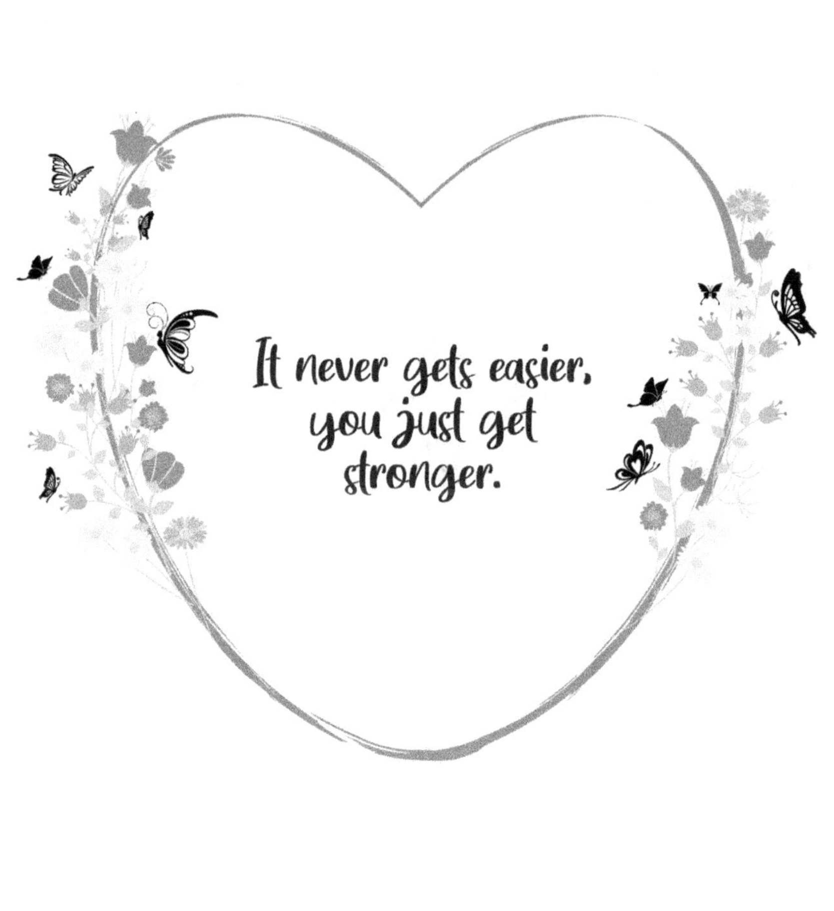
It never gets easier,
you just get
stronger.

Chapter 16: Get moving—exercise flushes toxins—a club I never planned on joining

After my surgery and radiation ended, I was blessed to be able to join a beautiful exercise facility within walking distance from my work. This facility also had a program for breast cancer thrivers.

Although my company has a wonderful on-site gym, I never used it. I was too busy for self-care. While I encouraged my team and others to take breaks and exercise, I never followed my own advice. How could my body detox from all of the stress it was under if I never moved? Guess what? It couldn't, and my body was becoming more toxic by the day.

Getting rid of toxins in the body will give you more energy. Here's another reason to exercise; exercise accelerates the detoxification process. Exercise pushes the blood to circulate more efficiently through the body, allowing nutrients to more easily reach all the organs and muscles. At the same time, exercise helps lymph fluids circulate through the body, which removes toxins and other harmful materials. When you exercise, you naturally take in more oxygen. To make room for the added oxygen, your cells kick out toxins that are taking up space. When you exercise properly, you build up a sweat and toxins are released through the pores of the skin.

Exercise benefits

Many research studies support the idea that exercising during cancer treatment helps you feel better. Some of the documented benefits include:

- Reduced depression and anxiety
- Increased energy and strength
- Reduced pain

Worried that it might not be safe? There's evidence to the contrary. For instance, when researchers reviewed 61 studies involving women with stage II breast cancer, they found that a combination of aerobic and resistance exercise was not only safe, it also improved health outcomes.

Other studies have found that exercise during treatment can actually change the tumor microenvironment and trigger stronger anti-tumor activity in your immune system. And very recent animal studies have found that exercise can lead to tumor reduction in rodents.

Physical activity also helps you manage your weight, which is an important cancer risk factor. In fact, research has linked being overweight or obese to an increased risk of many types of cancer, including endometrial, esophageal, liver, pancreas and breast cancers. There's also increasing evidence that being overweight may lead to a higher risk of cancer recurrence and even cancer-related death.

All those health benefits associated with exercise during cancer treatment. Sound good, right? So maybe it's time to get started.

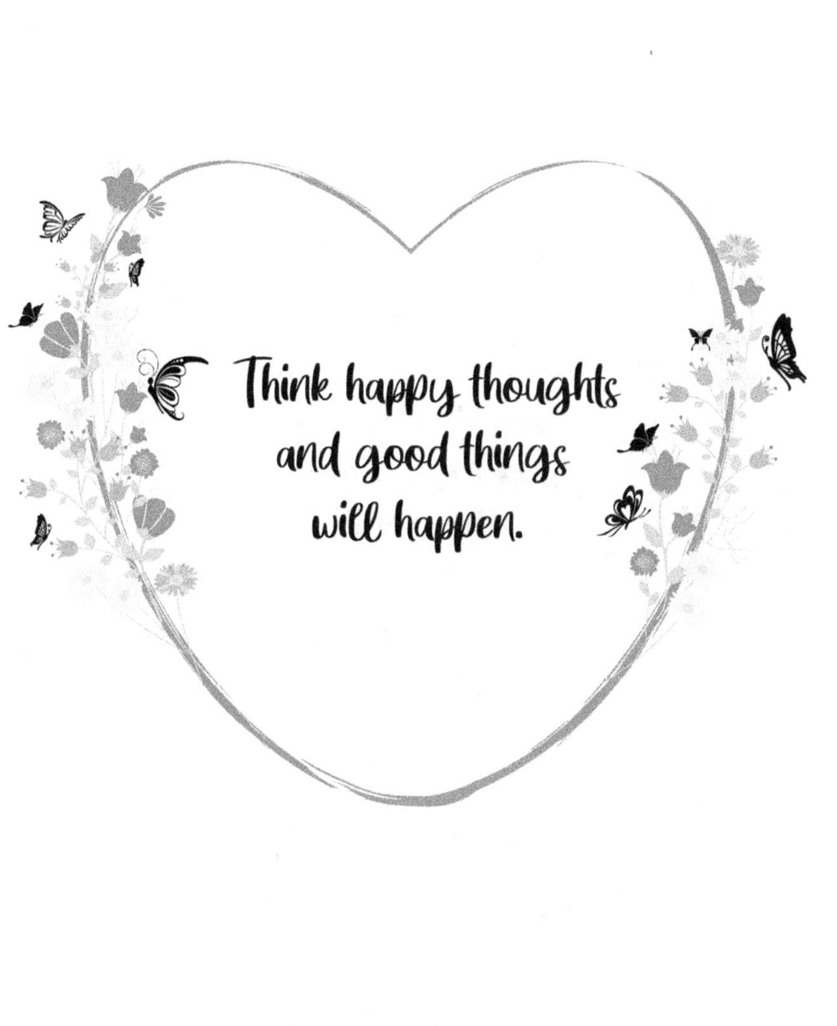

Think happy thoughts
and good things
will happen.

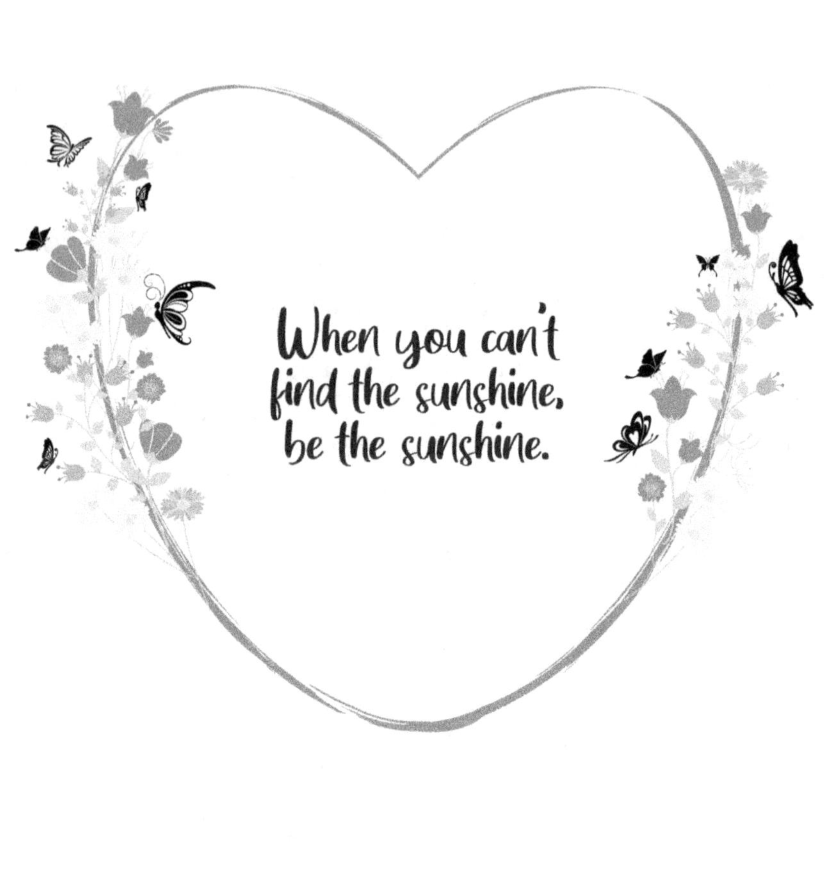

When you can't
find the sunshine,
be the sunshine.

Chapter 17: Fake it until you make it

Your mind is a powerful tool for healing.

Many times during my healing journey I would say out loud that I was healed and that all of my cancer cells were gone. I repeated the words "I am happy, healthy and never felt better." Most days this was true, but other times I was exhausted, sore and wanted to sleep. When I had hard days it never stopped me from saying positive affirmations to myself and looking into the future, seeing me playing with my grandkids and traveling the world with my husband. I believed I was well and thriving and each day my body became stronger.

In his book *You Are the Placebo* and in various videos, Dr. Joe Dispenza shared many stories of how each of us can turn our minds and bodies around to divine health. I believe we all have the ability to believe that our bodies can heal themselves. In my case it was my mind and God that healed me.

Before cancer I would complain about my ailments, but no longer. Each day I look out of my bedroom window, thank God for another day and believe that each day I am stronger and my body is healing and will fight to keep me well.

Please, please say positive things to yourself on a daily basis. It may sound odd, however, I believe your body and cells are listening. Even on days you don't feel your best find an affirmation that works for you and say it— just fake it until you make it!

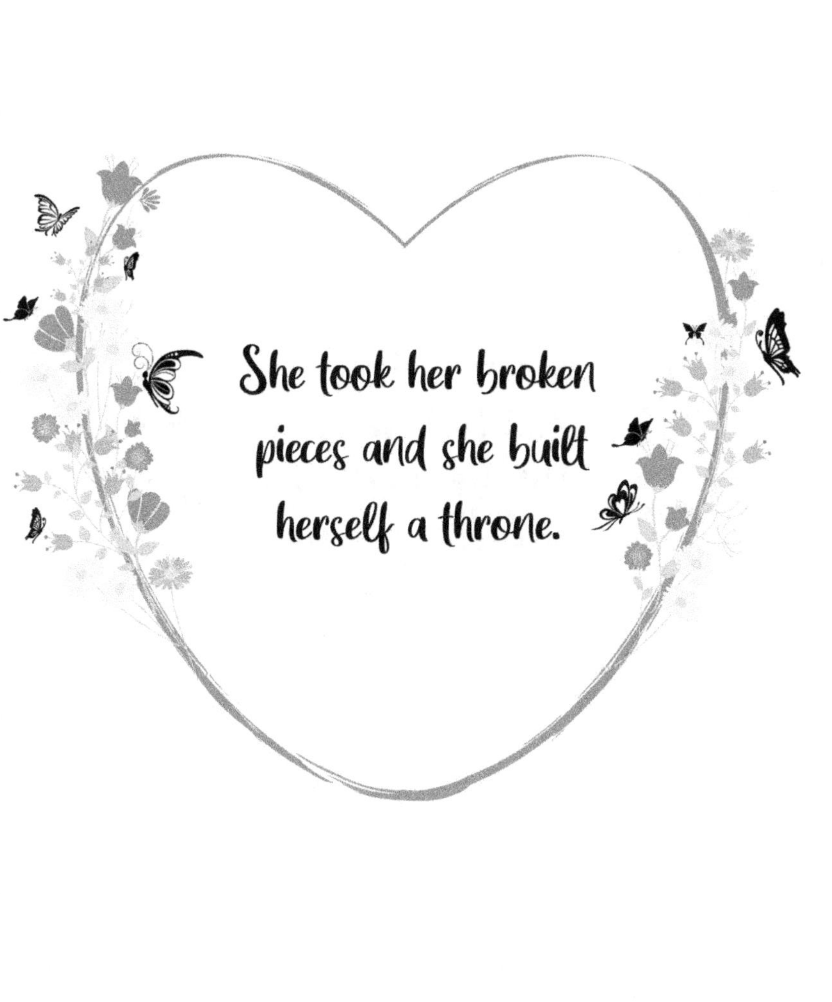

She took her broken
pieces and she built
herself a throne.

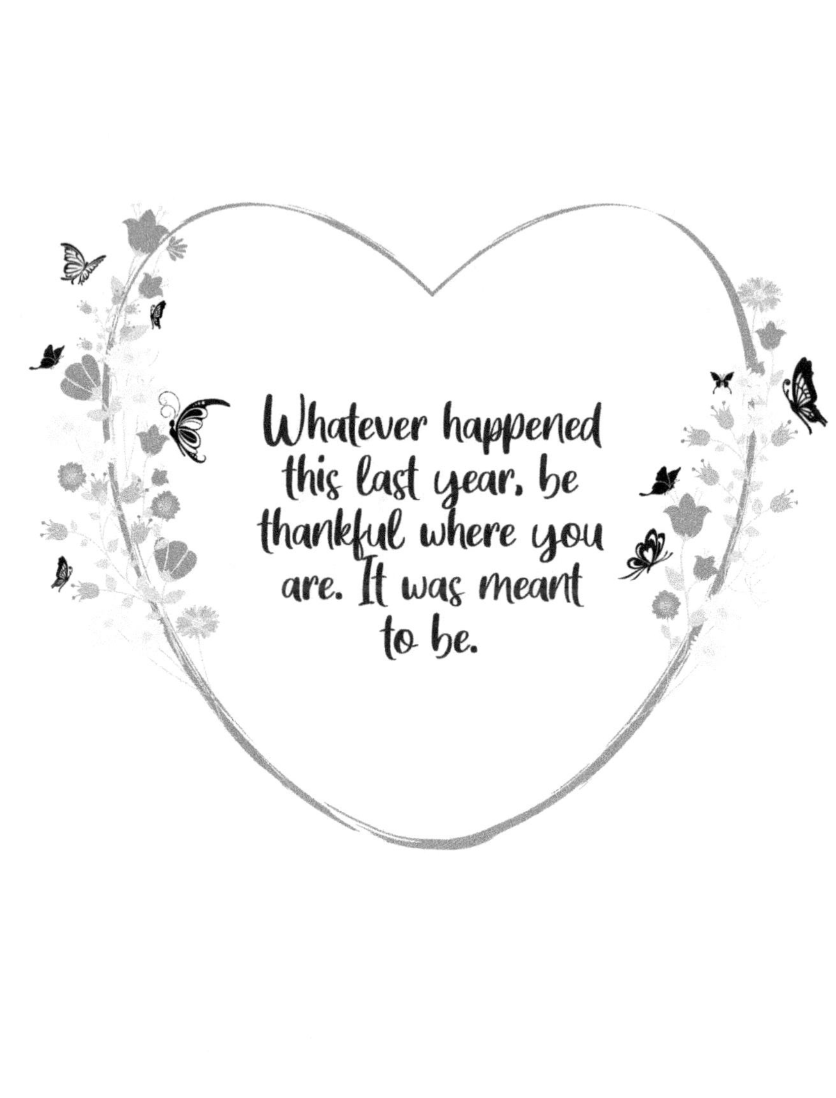
Whatever happened
this last year, be
thankful where you
are. It was meant
to be.

Chapter 18: Gratitude must be your new attitude

I use my Dear Lord journal that my best friend gave me the week of my diagnosis every night to write down all of my reasons to be grateful, no matter how small they might be—even if it's just the mere fact that I am alive to breathe! Gratitude can change your life because it makes you appreciate what you have rather than what you don't have. Gratitude can change your life because it is the single most powerful source of inspiration that any person can tap into if they simply just stop and pay attention to the simplistic beauty and miracle of life.

A transformational shift can occur when you become utterly grateful for everything in your life, even your problems. Having true gratitude for things has completely changed my life. I transformed from an ungrateful, never-took-time-to-smell-the-roses kind of person to having an appreciation for all things.

Whatever realm of thought you're living in, the importance of gratitude cannot be underestimated. There are specific reasons why gratitude can change your life, and if you listen to them and truly hear the message beyond the words, there are some incredible things that will begin to happen for you over time. Begin to have an ever-grateful attitude for what you have today, right now, in this very moment, rather than what you're lacking.

Gratitude shifts your focus

Gratitude is not just about being a positive person; having gratitude can change your life because it breathes positivity into everything you're doing. It's a monumental shift in focus, a new way of seeing things, one that involves a wild-eyed appreciation for the beauty of all things. You move from living in a state of lack to living in a state of sheer abundance in every possible way.

Still, this doesn't happen overnight; however, you can move from a negative state to a positive state by recounting all of the things that you have to be grateful for on a daily basis and writing them down. The key is to write it down. Writing makes it more real rather than an abstract concept living in your mind.

Being grateful makes you feel happier

One way that gratitude can change your life is by making you happier. Studies have confirmed that having gratitude does in fact make you feel happier. When we're grateful for things, it's a natural occurrence to be happier about life. You realize the things you have rather than the things you don't. It's far easier to go about your day in a state of appreciation when you're grateful than when you're not. Being grateful puts you into a state of abundance. It instills the belief that you're thankful for what you have, right now, in this very moment, rather than worrying about what you don't have or won't have at some future point in time.

Gratitude strengthens and enhances your faith
Gratitude can transform your life by strengthening and enhancing your faith. For me, it's my belief in God and the realization that I am truly and completely grateful for everything in my life, including all my problems.

Gratitude transforms your faith by instilling the belief that you're not alone and that whatever it is that you're going through, it will pass, and on the other end you'll emerge victorious. You'll search for opportunities because you realize that what you have truly is enough and that the focus must become helping others. That's when true spiritual enlightenment begins.

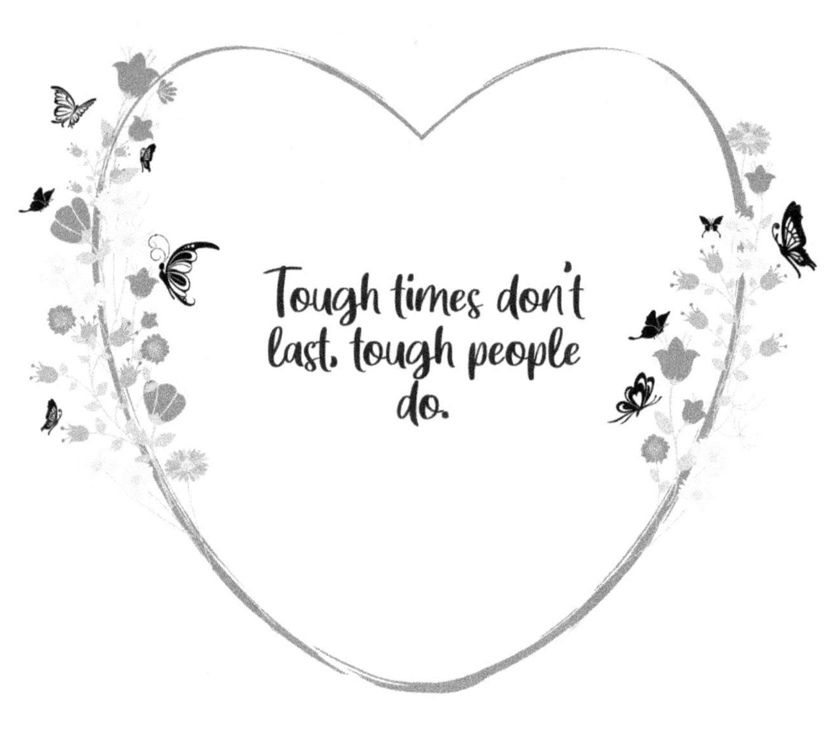

Tough times don't last, tough people do.

Chapter 19: The test results and the all clear

All cancer patients want to hear the words "You are all clear." I received those words in November 2019. This was my gift from God. I have the piece of paper that says this. I look at it often for encouragement. I had a tribe that got me through my darkest days, but my true healer who will keep me thriving until I am in my 90s is God. I will continue to look for His messages and share them with others.

I feel so blessed, healthy and full of energy. I would never go back to my past way of living. Everything has changed. I feel like a have a new life.

Below is a summary of the messages I learned. I pray that these help you in your healing journey to divine health.

Early detection is key. Please schedule your yearly breast exams on time.

A cancer diagnosis is terrifying. Find your small tribe on whom you can lean, to whom you can cry and with whom you can share how darn scared you are until you know your next steps. First in your tribe should be God.

Cancer does not grow overnight. You have time to research the best treatment options for you and to assemble the best team!

Look for the good in your cancer message. I promise you will find it.

Expand your tribe when you are ready. You will need their support and prayers.

Until you have your cancer tumor removed and examined along with the lymph nodes, it is difficult to know the exact makeup of your cancer and you cannot start to formulate your treatment plan. The initial biopsy is not always accurate!

Know your odds and listen to your gut!

Listen to your gut and heart. This is your body and mind—God is our healer.

Do what makes you smile during your treatments—music heals!

Smile at strangers—you may make a friend. Rest, rest, rest during radiation. Care for your skin a few times a day. Be sure the lotions and potions you use on your breast are organic and non-toxic.

You must clear your toxic emotions before you can fully heal.

Find your spiritual healers and pray!

Find a holistic dentist to remove your mercury fillings with the SMART method.

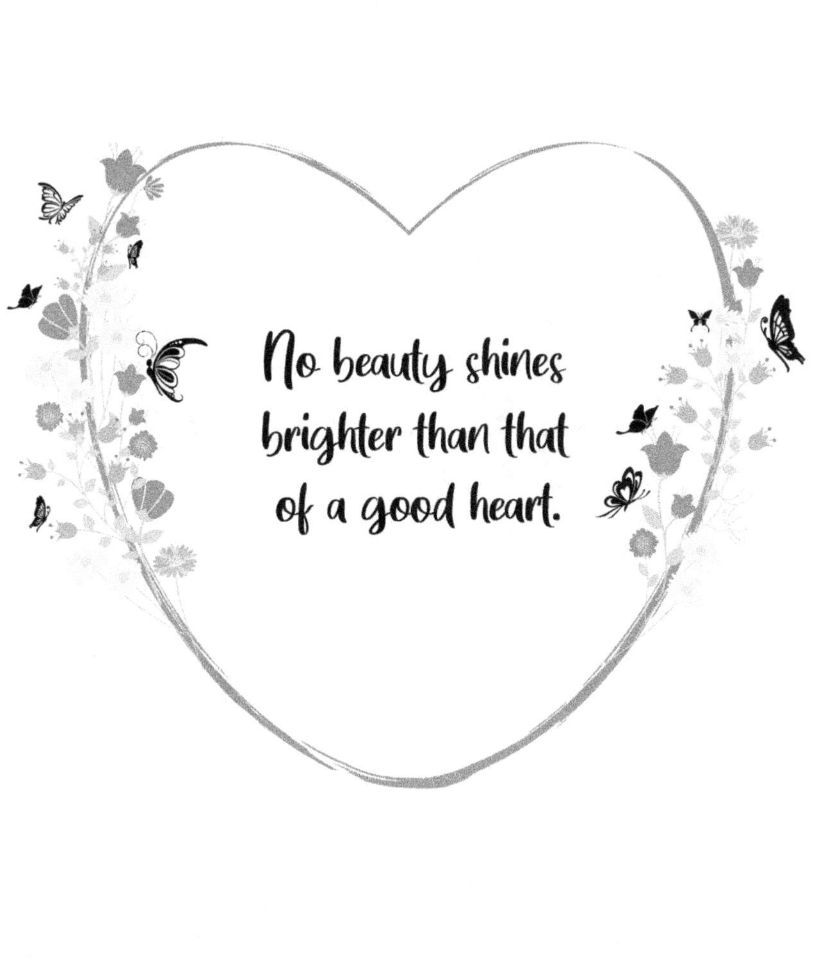

No beauty shines
brighter than that
of a good heart.

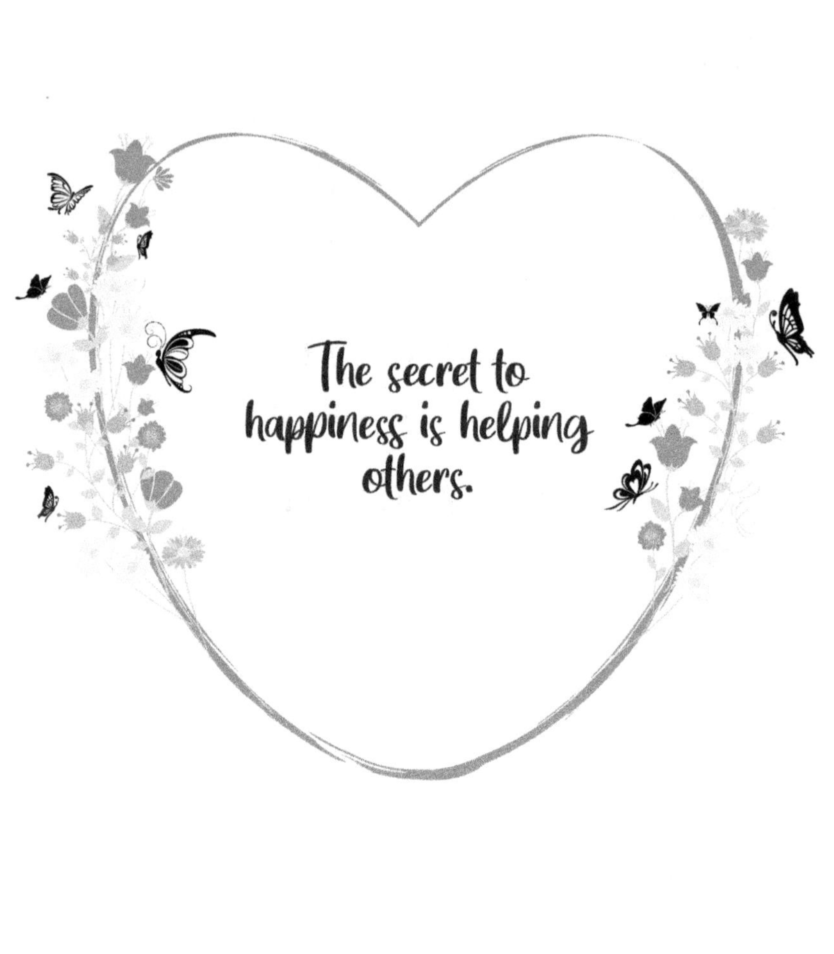
The secret to
happiness is helping
others.

Chapter 20: My reasons to thrive— be someone's miracle

I knew I was blessed beyond measure prior to my cancer diagnosis, but I was not grateful. In fact, I took my health and many other things, big and small, for granted. From the day I heard those terrifying words, I knew at that second I wanted to live. I wanted to live a long and healthy life. I begged God to give me the chance to change.

As a wife and mother, I want to live for my husband and children. Although my children are young adults, I want to be there to encourage them, love them and watch them blossom with their own families. My husband and I have a bucket list and amazing memories that need to be continued. My parents and my brother need their daughter and sister to be around. I am an aunt and daughter-in-law as well. It is obvious that one's would be a reason to live. However, I realized when I was healing that I also had a group of co-workers and friends who came forward to tell me how I have affected them, if even in some small way. One of my reasons to live and thrive is to make a difference, to be a role model for courage and gratefulness. I want to make even a tiny impact in someone's life. I read a great book by Joel Osteen and in his message he said, "Be someone's miracle." That is what I will strive to do.

During my healing journey, God sent an old high school friend to me who I hadn't spoken with in over 35 years. This beautiful woman is dealing with stage IV colon cancer and didn't have much of a support system. I tried to provide her hope and encouragement through her journey. She sent me a lovely note that I will treasure. The message that God sent me was, "Even though you are going through your healing journey, focus on helping someone else who may need hope."

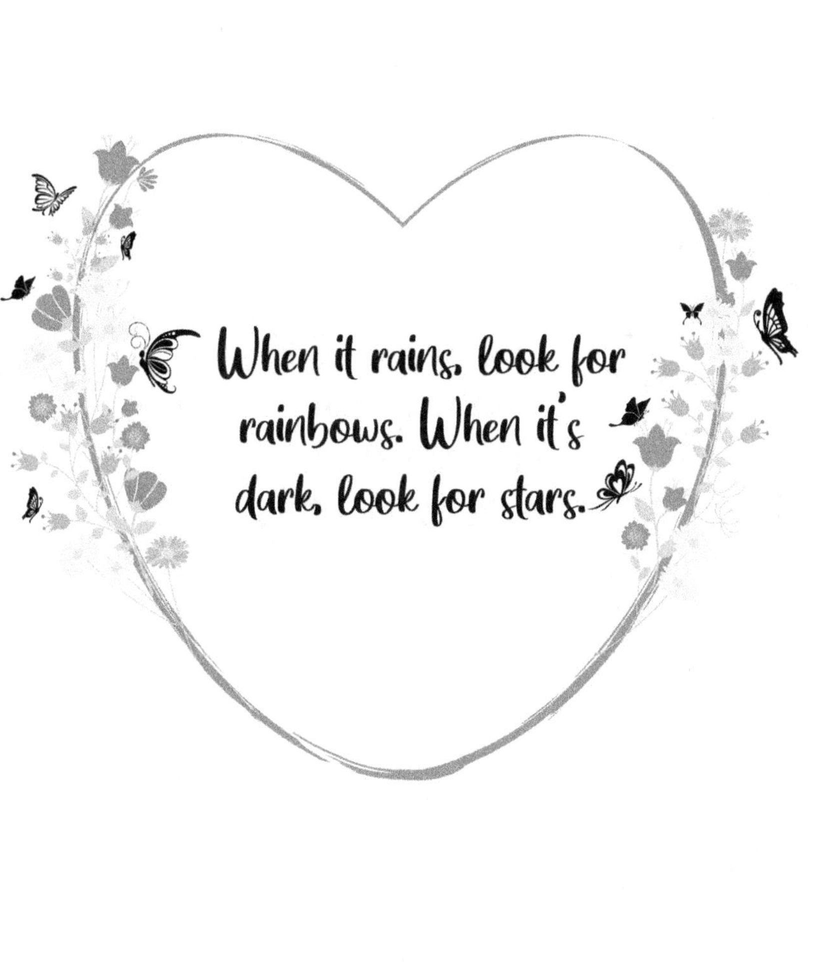

When it rains, look for
rainbows. When it's
dark, look for stars.

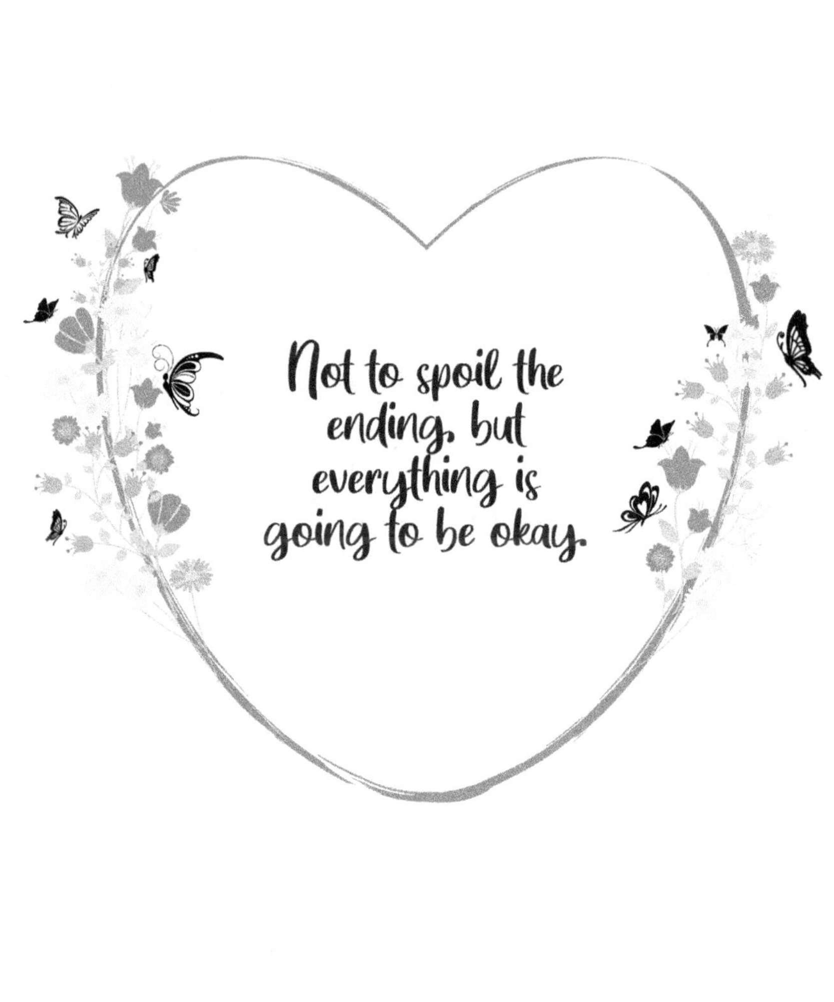
Not to spoil the
ending, but
everything is
going to be okay.

Appendix: Recommended Reading

- *My Time with God: Renewed in His Presence Daily*, Joyce Meyer
- *Chris Beat Cancer: A Comprehensive Plan for Healing Naturally*, Chris Wark
- *Radical Remission: Surviving Cancer Against All Odds*, Kelly A Turner
- *Heal Breast Cancer Naturally*, Dr. Véronique Desaulniers
- *You Are the Placebo*, Joe Dispenza
- *How to Starve Cancer*, Jane McLelland
- *Knockout*, Suzanne Somers
- *The Cancer Revolution: A Groundbreaking Program to Reverse and Prevent Cancer*, Dr. Leigh Erin Connealy
- *Shine Beyond Cancer: 7 Steps To Living A Better Life*, Lisa Dimond and Marc Slugh
- *My Way : Following the cancer brick road, from diagnosis to all clear naturally in 5 months . . .*, Dee Mani
- *Super Attractor*, Gabrielle Bernstein

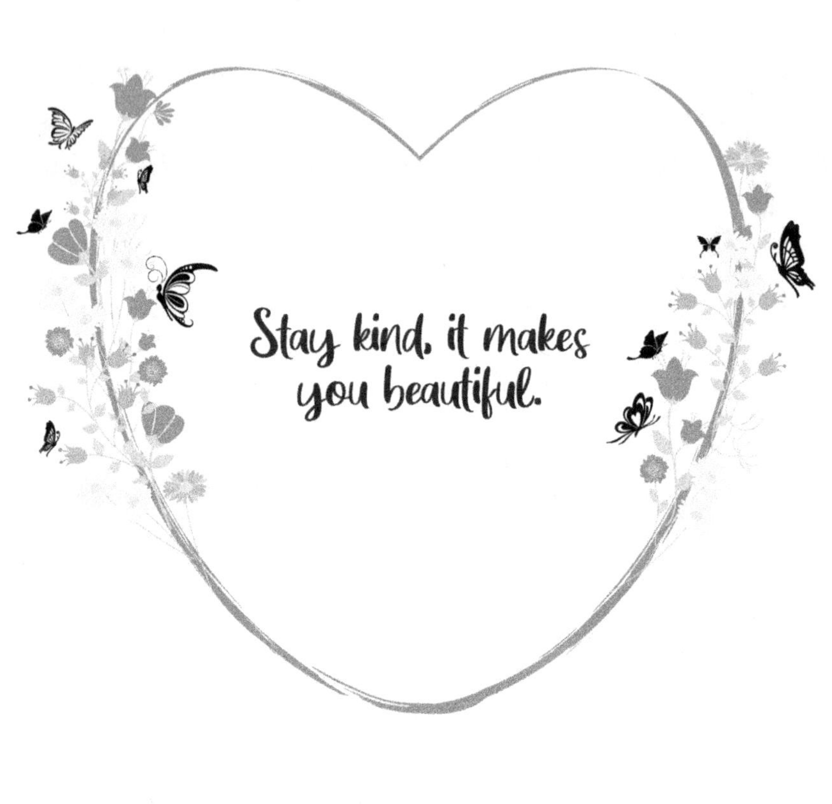
Stay kind, it makes
you beautiful.

Corinna Alandt resides in northern California with her husband, two adult children and rescue Poochon dog. She has an executive position with a Fortune 500 financial services company.

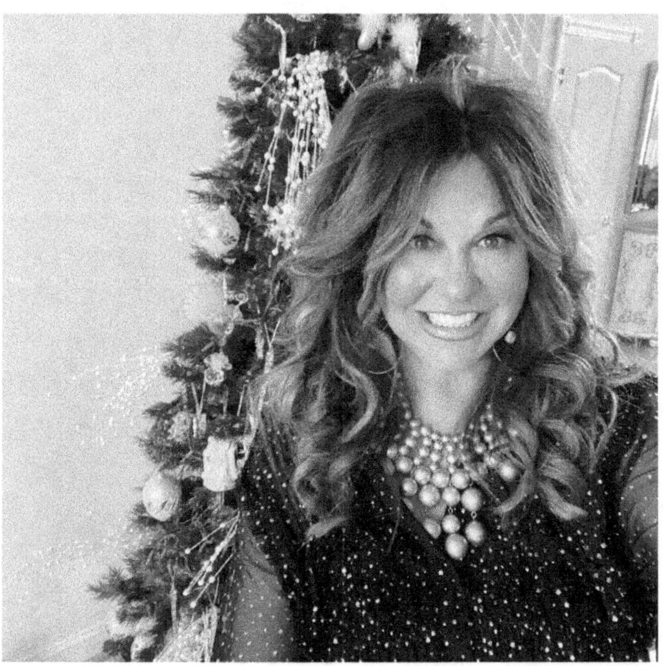